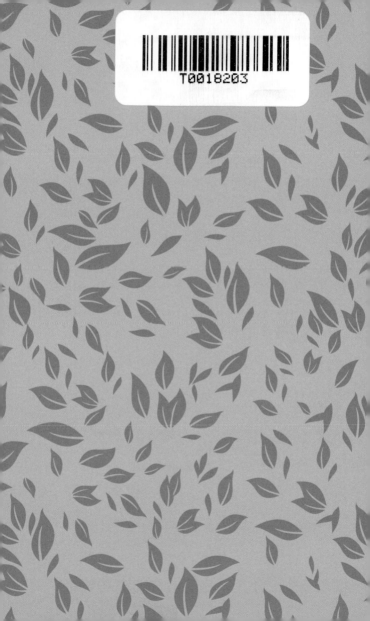

T0018203

HERBALISM

HERBALISM
PLANTS AND POTIONS THAT HEAL

ADRIAN WHITE

SIRIUS

ACKNOWLEDGEMENTS

Much thanks to the herbalists, friends, experts, growers, chefs and other specialists who contributed and shared their own creations to this book for others to learn and benefit from in their own health and healing. Most thanks of all to the ancient and ancestral peoples the world over who developed and kept this lore for us to use and benefit from.

AUTHOR'S WEB SITE:

IowaHerbalist.com

All illustrations courtesy of Shutterstock

SIRIUS

This edition published in 2022 by Sirius Publishing, a division of Arcturus Publishing Limited,
26/27 Bickels Yard, 151–153 Bermondsey Street,
London SE1 3HA

ISBN: 978-1-3988-2094-4
AD008727UK

Printed in China

CONTENTS

INTRODUCTION

HISTORY OF HERBALISM

L ong before modern medicine, there was herbalism – though not as long ago as you might think. In the Western world, and in the United States specifically, herbal medicine only went out of vogue as recently as the 19th century. Before that, the use of herbs was the dominant form of healing.

Herbal medicine still dominates healthcare on the planet; many Westerners just don't know it. It is eclipsed by pharmaceuticals, hospitals, allopathy, and more conventional methods that have been scientifically tested and sold as more effective than simple plants in our everyday lives. **According to the World Health Organization (WHO), 80% of people around the globe still use herbal or botanical medicines as part of their primary healthcare**. This includes people in developing countries for whom modern medicine may not be an option, along with indigenous, cultural or ethnic groups holding on to traditional plant-based healing practices from centuries past. It also includes mainstream medical practices that have either always integrated – or are now rapidly integrating – herbal medicine as part of everyday treatment in non-Western parts of the world. Some examples include Traditional Chinese Medicine (TCM), Ayurvedic practices in Asia, and some European countries where prescriptions for herbs are again being approved by doctors. Last but not least, it includes herbal practitioners, home herbalists, kitchen witches and country doctors who have held on to herbal traditions left over from the ancient Western world.

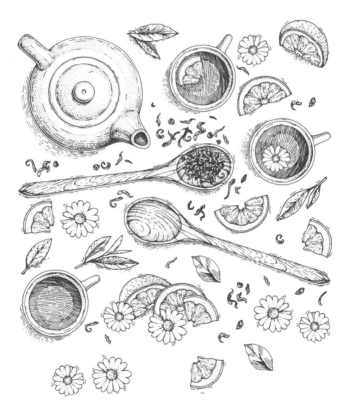

So why is herbalism still around, if modern medicine seems to 'work better'? Because herbs have always worked, and still do – just in a different way, and one that has been lost to popular Western understanding. Westerners now have a chance to look at the world of herbalism with fresh eyes. Westerners like myself can establish our own herbal traditions in a new and modern way, while nodding to our own ancestors' use of plant medicines and nutrition first and foremost, while respecting the contributions other racial and indigenous traditions have mastered, protected and survived with for centuries. It is important to note that some contributions from minorities have an undeniably bloody history that can no longer go unmentioned in herbal works penned by the non-indigenous and non-POC, as we work to decolonize herbalism understanding.

***

My first brush with herbal healing took place while travelling in a remote area of Ecuador, in the Andes, where many people live to be over 100. I didn't go there to learn about herbal healing, but one day I was injured. With medical services and hospitals a half-hour away by horseback and an hour away by bus, it was my first time experiencing what medicine was like for the 80% of the world that relies on botanical medicine. I was quick to join that statistic afterward: locals showed me how to identify a plant (distantly related to black pepper and kava kava) that could be boiled into a dark tea for pulling out and cleansing infections. Long story short, without the help of that herb – and the natives' knowledge of it and generosity in sharing it with me – I could have very well lost my foot.

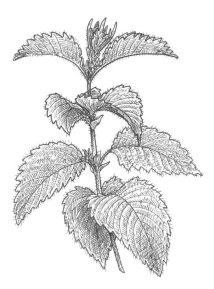

I've seen herbs work in dramatic ways, and in much subtler yet still powerfully effective ways. Some herbs, like that South American one, work like a tsunami, while others work slowly, over time, until one day you realize that some aspect of your health has been restored and transformed. I've seen herbs work quickly to help symptoms like allopathic medicine (think Ibuprofen for inflammation, for example) but also provide the body with vitamins, minerals, antioxidants and phytonutrients that can help prevent issues. I've felt my energy return and anxiety fade from being burnt out at a highly demanding, stressful job after weeks of consuming stinging nettle daily. I've felt soothed and restored with a simple cup of lemon balm tea right before a job interview when my stomach was in knots. I've seen lion's mane stop tremors and spasms; I've seen remedies like agrimony settle allergic reactions, an overactive liver and even an asthma attack in seconds. I've seen estrogenic herbs, like angelica, rid a person of terrible acne.

The more incredible thing about what I've said above: these are personal experiences, and are not necessarily health claims (though herbs can and definitely do work scientifically and predictably). I encourage you to try out herbs (safely) in the contexts for which they have been scientifically researched, as well as for their 'folk' uses accumulated over hundreds if not thousands of years. However, as some practised herbalists will tell you, plants can form very special – almost spiritual and definitely near magickal – relationships with those who get taken up with them. You could even say that herbs get taken up with those who use them, too, playing a mysterious role in their effects. While this is true for myself and many other seasoned herbalists out there, I obviously have to recommend that you only experiment and use herbs in this way safely and at your discretion; any reported benefits from approaches like these are completely subjective. And, on a scientific (not just spiritual or spooky) level, certain herbs work better for some people, but not so well for others.

Novice herbalists find themselves attracted to a certain arsenal of healing herbs for their own uses, based on their own experiences with them. And the beauty – and magick – of it all is that every herbalist's methodology, apothecary, 'medicine cabinet', 'materia medica' or whatever you call it will be different. **The herbs you will learn about in this book are by no means all that's out there, or even considered a 'classic' list.** These are simply the ones I've taken a shine to, which have worked for me, and which

I've also researched on a scientific basis. As a white Westerner, I have decided to choose predominantly Western herbal remedies that reflect my European ancestry, with a few exceptions like aloe vera (from Africa and the Middle East), lion's mane (East Asia) and sumac (Native North America) that I couldn't help but feel a personal call to honour and write about – mostly

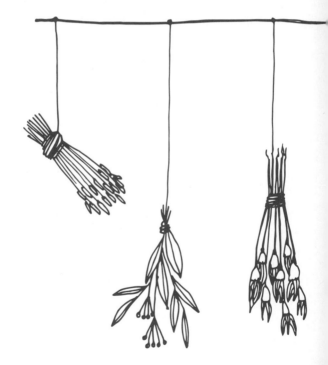

because of how efficaciously and powerfully I have experienced them in my own life.

This book is an introductory reference for those who may not only be interested in simple herbalism for self-care at home, but may also eventually be interested in building their own apothecaries, formulating herbal preparations, creating products, and digging into the

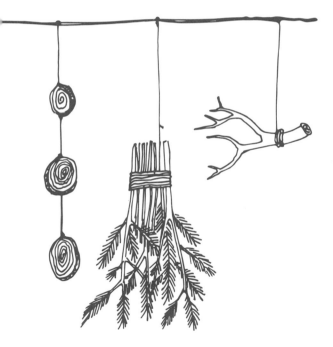

nitty-gritty of actual, practical healing using botanicals. Here is a quick guide to using this book as a reference:

For quick reference, first peruse the Monographs section (profiles of certain plants) if you wish to get acquainted with very detailed examples of healing herbs. Then, cross-reference to the Harvesting and Preparations sections. Each profile will indicate how these are harvested or prepared, and tell you which page to refer to.

For specific or specialized approaches to harvesting or preparing herbs, check out the

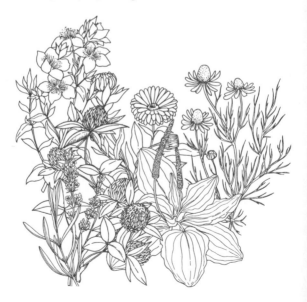

unique recipes or preparations, contributed by working herbal practitioners, growers, food experts and home herbalists, and given under each monograph.

Don't know where to start? Skip to the Constitutions, Energetics, and Tastes of Herbs sections to learn more about yourself, health states and a quick way to categorize what herbs can do – and to help you figure out which ones you may be partial to.

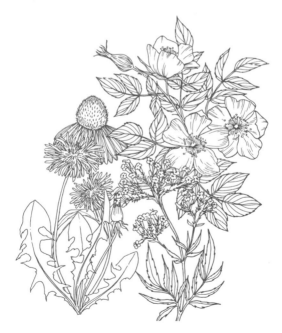

Read this book cover to cover. There's nothing wrong with that.

There are an untold number of medicinal plants on this planet. The world of herbalism is full of endless exploration. The exciting part is that the learning process never really ends. Even if you become a self-proclaimed herbalist expert – and complete multiple training programmes, apprenticeships, read tons of books, research regularly and attend every herbal school you can think of – there are still new plants to get acquainted with and try, and new healing experiences to be had in your daily life. I hope this book is a fun first step closer to that.

DISCLAIMER

The information in this book is not meant to prescribe, diagnose, promote or make claims about any natural or herbal remedies and what they can do. It is not recommended to use this book as a replacement for professional healthcare or the supervision of a doctor. If you are diagnosed with a health condition or dealing with serious health symptoms, please contact your doctor or another health professional right away.

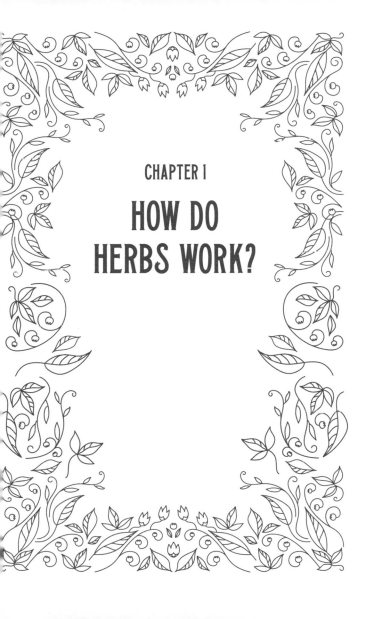

CHAPTER 1

HOW DO HERBS WORK?

Curiosity is what sparks the interest of every novice herbalist. The appeal of caring for and healing one's health at home, with the help of plants, is hard to resist – and the results can be astonishing, empowering, even life-changing. If this makes the use of herbs for health sound incredible, that's because it is. Or, more accurately, it can be, if you learn how herbs work, their proper role in your life and your health, their limitations, and how to manage your expectations of them.

There are two sides to every coin. As you try herbs and get acquainted with them, you'll no doubt have some powerful experiences. And you will come to learn the limits of their effectiveness. Plants have tons of potential for health, but newcomers to herbalism can project their hopes and wishes on herbs and then be disappointed – especially if mainstream medicine has failed them or if there is a belief that herbs work just like conventional medicines, like pharmaceuticals. Some newcomers may have been exposed to the false belief in the effects of 'fad herbs', false advertising around herb effects, transforming herbs into new 'superfoods', or the idea of 'miracle cures' or magic-bullet remedies.

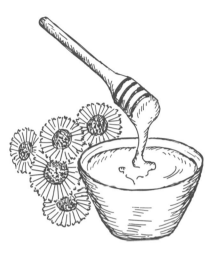

Herbalism is not a secret, untapped underground healing method adjacent to mainstream medicine. It is not somehow better or even the 'true' form of healthcare, self-care or nutrition we all need. It is just different, an alternative or complement; that is why herbalism is often placed in the category of 'alternative' or 'complementary' medicine, though it ought to be more *foundational* than modern medicine. Herbalism is a simpler, more natural approach to taking care of health and the body that the world (mostly the white Western world) has long lost – replaced by conventional medicine, leaving modern healing quite one-sided. According to some ancient health traditions – especially in Asia, though also elsewhere – human beings may have been healthier in the past compared to the average person today thanks in part to herbs; especially when they were consumed daily, much like a food, prepared in food, used as a seasoning, or as a daily beverage (like tea).

Though they shouldn't replace mainstream medicine, the impact herbs and foods can have – and have had – on health shouldn't be underestimated. **We do indeed have proof of what is lost when healthful plants are taken from a people and replaced with synthetic medicines and a processed Western diet** – such as in the case of indigenous and minority groups showing worse health outcomes after losing access to ancestral foods and remedies due to colonization. Groups that have lost their foodways, including herbs, have also lost their most important medicines. Because of this, and as modern research on herbal remedies continues to catch up with the empirical knowledge of master herbal practitioners centuries ago, it's also becoming clear that plant therapies shouldn't be an 'alternative' or 'complement' – they ought to be integrated into primary health and self-care.

❦ Herbs as holistic healers

Understanding herbs and how they work best, in one sense, can be explained with the word 'holistic'. **Holistic** means that a remedy works for the *whole* body and the *entire* disease, bodily system, or imbalance. It is not just an independent issue or symptom – this idea is called **allopathic healthcare** (or **allopathy**, the approach to health that currently dominates conventional mainstream medicine). Today, the most advanced treatments involve pharmaceutical pills, chemical treatments, radiation, surgery and other interventions, some of which can eradicate illnesses like cancer. But on the whole, allopathy is designed to suppress and get rid of symptoms only, not the disease itself (and sometimes at the expense of other health aspects or bodily symptoms).

Herbs, on the other hand, are full of health-specific phytochemicals and antioxidants that enhance the health of the entire body, if not targeted organs and bodily systems, in most cases along with vitamins and minerals that our bodies may need. The holistic effect is that herbs – as supplements, teas, tinctures, extracts and more – can enhance the health and strength of the body, allowing it to cope with the illness or imbalance directly, thus helping reduce both the symptoms *and* the disease.

❧ Herbs as functional foods (food as medicine)

Herbs as holistic remedies can step powerfully into your healthcare when taken daily, and not just in supplement form. When you learn about famous healing herbs like garlic, ginger or turmeric, their potential as healing foods when eaten regularly is fairly obvious – especially since many are already well-established as culinary seasonings or spices. Thinking of herbs as functional foods, or 'food as medicine', can also help one use them properly for boosting health – whether that's immune health, respiratory health, liver health, cardiovascular health, brain health or any other system (though skin health, topical health or wound healing are entirely different approaches). The important emphasis with 'food' is *daily* use. For example: taking milk thistle for liver health, or for a detoxifying benefit, may have an effect if taken in one sitting. But the benefits are better by far when milk thistle is part of your daily diet.

When looking at herbs as holistic supplements, or incorporating them into the diet as foods, this is where they differ greatly from over-the-counter pills or prescription drugs. Taking certain herbs

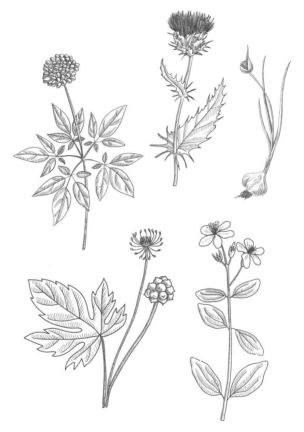

only one time, or every once in a while, won't have the desired effect. Many need to be consumed daily, for a long time, and their overall benefit is a gradual one – just like taking a vitamin every day.

That said, some botanicals – even in small doses, for one-time use – have been known to do rather impressive things.

✂ Herbs as homeopathic remedies

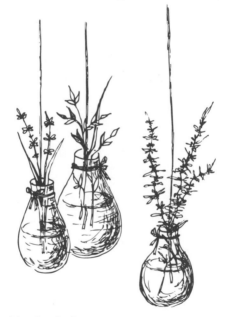

Some older herbalist practices work under the concept of 'homeopathy', the idea that 'like treats like' when it comes to illness. This book won't examine this approach too much since it is food- and nutrition-oriented, and can involve highly toxic and dangerous plants. But, since many herbalists use this principle – and some common herbal products are indeed homeopathic preparations – it deserves a mention, especially since many herbalists work with the modality (not just with humans, but with animals too) and report great success. (Herbal monograph of agrimony, found on p. 99, includes a formulation recipe and a nod to homeopathy and homeopathic flower essences.)

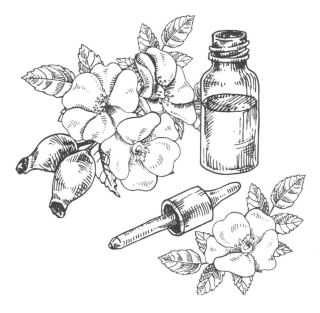

Homeopathy involves extremely small doses of a herbal medicine – sometimes as little as a few drops of tincture or extract – and can have profound effects on the body. Sometimes, homeopathic preparations don't technically contain any ingredients of the herb itself, only its spirit or 'essence' (such as flower essences) captured in a water solution. Herbal ingredients or essences in homeopathic remedies are often chosen because large amounts of them could *cause* the same illness or symptom it treats. For example, foxglove is used in extremely low doses for heart health. In normal or large doses, it could *cause* heart conditions, or even heart failure. (Sound dangerous? We nevertheless have homeopathy to thank for some very effective blood-pressure medications currently in use, which contain compounds from the foxglove plant.)

The idea is that extremely small doses can do just enough to trigger the body to cure those very same symptoms. But for the beginner herbalist, safety is a big consideration. That said, many herbalists (including myself) experience great and surprising success – sometimes immediate effects – from safe, low-dose botanicals. Herbs can work in mysterious ways.

🌿 When herbs act like mainstream medicine

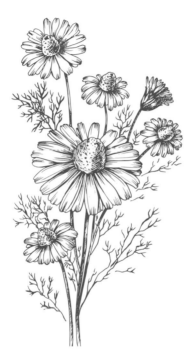

There are certain herbs that work a lot like mainstream allopathic remedies – not unlike over-the-counter medicines. Some digestive herbs, such as angelica, lemon balm or hops, can have an immediate effect – soothing an upset stomach or cramps, for example. Have you sipped a ginger ale while nauseous? The effects are immediate. Medical cannabis (and CBD) is another example of herbs working like allopathic medicine, soothing not only nausea but also nerve pain (including, in some cases, nerve pain that pharmaceutical painkillers can't touch).

Anti-anxiety and sedative effects are also notable. Who hasn't sipped some chamomile tea to feel a sense of relaxation within moments? (If you haven't, go and make some; see pp. 136–139 for tea recipes featuring chamomile.) Though a little less common, many of us have tried valerian root (pp. 171–176) to find sleep coming on that little bit sooner.

Topical use and minor wound treatment are also great uses for herbs in an allopathic sense: aloe for minor burn treatment, pine as an antimicrobial for superficial wounds, and plantain for bug bites. These are only a few examples of herbal treatments that have immediate and powerful effects.

Herbs, spirituality, ritual and magickal uses

Almost all plants – whether used as functional foods, holistic remedies or like allopathic treatments – also have spiritual uses. These spiritual (or in some cases, magickal) uses are defined by the cultures that first learned to work with and master their uses, whether medicinal, spiritual or both.

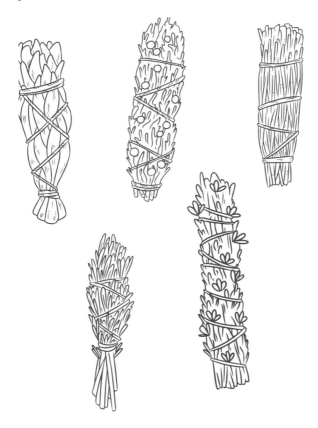

In some belief systems, the spiritual benefits are experienced alongside the more 'medicinal' effects in whatever form they are taken. For example: in many cultures, consuming garlic protects not only against colds and flu, but also negative or unwanted spiritual influence from others. It is protective both within and without. Mugwort, another example, can be consumed as a tea for sedative effects, but also to open up spiritual abilities and enhance dream life. It can be smudged or burned like incense for the same spiritual effects, and can create a protective or cleansed space, much like the Native American white sage (but a European variant).

CHAPTER 2

BASIC HERBAL PREPARATIONS

The following recipes are ideal for home use and self-care. However, professional herbalists in clinical settings (and retail product craft makers) are encouraged to follow far more precise scientific calculations, alchemy, measurements and ratios in their practice, to get the most health benefits and potency out of their products. For that, I cannot recommend Richo Cech's book, *Making Plant Medicine*, enough. But, for the home health needs of just about anyone else, these basic recipes will do just fine.

Home herbalism, or cottage herbalism (or kitchen-witchin', as I like to call it), has been around for so long that I could hardly call the following how-to's anything close to a recipe, let alone a *signature* recipe; they are just one way to do things.

❧ Teas, Infusions, and Decoctions

Nothing is more synonymous with herbs and herbal healing than tea. Sipping herbal tea is the first encounter many have with herbs – not only with their flavour but their benefits and effects. Tea can be simple or complex. But, in the grand scheme of herbal preparations, it's almost always a mostly easy process to make teas, infusions or decoctions – the latter being teas made of 'tougher' herbal materials like bark, roots, twigs, or hard-skinned fungi. (More on these later.)

SIMPLE TEA RECIPE

While it's true that you can make tea out of any herb, a simple tea brings out the best in fresh, leafy herbs, fruits or flowers, especially a botanical's flavours and fragile constituents. That said, there's no reason not to enjoy a quick tea of herbal roots, bark and the like. These won't be nearly as potent or, in some cases, as flavourful as a decoction, but that doesn't mean they're not enjoyable or healthy.

STEP 1 – Bring water to a boil.
STEP 2 – In the meantime, ready a mug or teapot with the tea amounts you wish to use. Most herbs make an excellent tea when you use 1–3 tablespoons (approx. 2g to 6g) of herbal material per cup measurement, or average mug size full of hot water. (Obviously, make sure to boil and prepare ample water.)

Herbal material can be either measured teabag amounts (store-bought or handmade) or placed into an infuser in your vessel of choice.
STEP 3 – Pour boiled water over tea in your teacup, mug, pot, infuser or other vessel. Let it

steep for at least 5 minutes. Sip and enjoy while still hot, and flavour lightly with lemon juice, honey or any other flavourful or health-boosting addition you like, and experience the benefits. **Make as many cups as needed until the desired effect is achieved, or enjoy 1-2 cups daily for long-term nutritive benefits (first, be sure to check 'Warnings Before Use' with any herb you make tea from in this book).**

HERBAL INFUSION (OR COMPRESS)

All teas are infusions; they're one and the same. In my own personal practice, however, I tend to label infusions as stronger herbal teas, with more specific medicinal purposes owing to their stronger nature, of course. Infusions don't always need to be taken internally. If you want to make a herbal compress (for topical use, such as minor burns or wounds), prepare an infusion. A compress, or wash (for wounds), can be used for superficial cuts, skin issues and the like.

Or, like a tea, you can simply sip an infusion for a stronger bout of effects than from regular herbal tea. Most herbalists also tend to make higher amounts of infusions: either for multiple compresses, or for drinking regularly over several days (refrigerating and/or re-boiling it, of course).

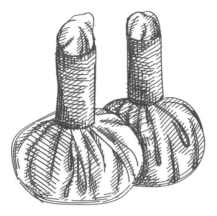

STEP 1 – Bring water to a boil.
STEP 2 – In the meantime, ready a large teapot or other stovetop pot with the infusion amounts you wish to use. These will be a higher ratio than teas. My personal ratio for a very strong tea infusion is ½–1 cup herb (dried or fresh) per 3.8 litres of water.
STEP 3 – Obviously, a teabag or infuser is not going to cut it for a strong infusion made in plentiful amounts (though large infusers can and do exist). I place all raw herbal material straight into the pot of boiling water, stir it in, and turn off the heat.
STEP 4 – Let the infusion steep for at least 10 minutes – some herbalists say at least 30

minutes, but there are no hard-and-fast rules. For a very potent brew, turn the pot on low instead of completely off, letting the herbs infuse for another hour.

STEP 5 – Once it reaches the desired strength, pour the infusion through a strainer into yet another clean stovetop pot to remove the herbal material. Pour into a cup (or multiple cups) as needed; flavour, sip and enjoy. **Make as many cups as needed until the desired effect is achieved, or enjoy 1–2 cups daily for long-term nutritive benefits (first, be sure to check 'Warnings Before Use' with any herb you make tea from in this book).**

You may also leave an infusion on low heat to enjoy multiple cups. Or turn off the heat, refrigerate, then reheat and enjoy later (ideally, infusions should be reheated and consumed within a week).

For using as a compress or wash, let the infusion cool. Then, using a clean cloth, apply the liquid to the area as many times as needed, or until the infusion is gone.

DECOCTIONS

Decoctions are reserved for the toughest herbal ingredients such as roots, bark, twigs and resilient fungi (e.g. reishi mushrooms, which are not explored in this book). The herbal materials don't steep. Instead, they are boiled for a long period of time, sometimes with water replenished or replaced as levels get lower. Like infusions, decoctions can be used for topical purposes in the form of a compress, too.

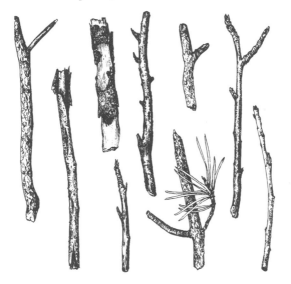

STEP 1 – Bring water to a boil in a large stovetop pot.
STEP 2 – Unlike teas or infusions, decoctions are made by putting the herbal material straight

into the boiling water. I use the same ratio for decoctions as with infusions (roughly ½–1 cup herb per 3.8 litres of water). Place the herbal material in the pot, either before the water comes to a boil or as soon as it starts to boil.

STEP 3 – Turn the boil down to a simmer, and let the herb infuse for between 1 and 2 hours. This helps extract constituents from the tougher herbal ingredients. One hour should produce a good decoction – however, you can decoct for much longer, and some herbalists even let it warm overnight, like a stew (ensuring that there is enough water, of course!).

STEP 4 – However long you choose to decoct, always make sure to stay nearby and keep an eye on the process. If the water begins to get low – or at a level lower than the herbal matter – add more, and let it continue to simmer. This is especially crucial if you decide to make a decoction overnight.

STEP 5 – Once it is to your liking, pour the decoction through a strainer into yet another clean stovetop pot or stainless-steel bowl, to remove the herbal material. Pour into a cup (or multiple cups) as needed; flavour, sip and enjoy. **Make as many cups as needed until the desired effect is achieved, or enjoy 1–2 cups daily for long-term nutritive benefits (first, be sure to**

check 'Warnings Before Use' with any herb you make tea from in this book).

As with an infusion, you can keep a decoction on a low heat to enjoy multiple cups. Or turn off the heat, refrigerate, then reheat and enjoy later (like infusions, decoctions should be consumed within a week).

For using as a compress, let the decoction cool. Then, using a clean cloth, apply the liquid to the area as many times as needed, or until the decoction is gone.

INFUSED OILS

Why make an infused oil? There are a couple of reasons. Before making a salve, you will need to make an infused oil. But not all infused oils necessarily need to be made into salves. Oils can also be used on their own, topically, just like salves for healing purposes; they can also be delightful when used in the kitchen – garlic-infused oil comes to mind (though less so for a topical salve).

Infused oils can be made with either fresh or dried herbs, a single herb or a combination of herbs. **Some herbalists follow tight ratios of herbs to oil, but generally, one part herbal matter to three parts oil is a good balance, and has worked for me**. Fresh infusions are favoured for salve-making, while dried herbs are preferable for culinary infused oils. This is because fresh herbs can impart water into the oil and increase the risk of pathogenic contamination if taken internally – which is why it is best to conserve these for topical use only.

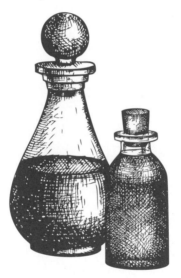

There are both crude and sophisticated ways to make infused oils, and the more sophisticated ways take more time, money and tools than a beginning herbalist may possess. Fortunately, the basic ways of creating herb-infused oils (not essential oils, to be clear –

these require distillation) are nearly as good for home use.

Note on proper oils: If you have standards of health and purity for the oils you buy for cooking, you'll want to have the same for your herb-infused oils. Be sure to purchase chemical-free, unrefined and otherwise pure choices.

• *Sun-Infused Oil*

STEP 1 – Place a measurement of herbs (single or multiple) in a clean jar that can be shut with an airtight lid (a standard large canning jar works great).

STEP 2 – Pour oil over the herbs in the jar. Make sure they are completely covered – this will ensure a good infusion.

STEP 3 – Place the jar in a sunny spot (such as a windowsill) to absorb a good amount of heat from the sun daily. South-facing windows are best since they'll ensure the best exposure and warmth – and it's important to make sure the container is tightly closed.

STEP 4 – Let the oil infuse in this way for about a week. Feel free to check on it and stir the mixture occasionally.

STEP 5 – After the week is over, strain the oil with a fine strainer or piece of cheesecloth into another container (you may use an empty, cleaned cooking-oil bottle; be sure to label it). Store in a cool, dry place and make sure the bottle or container is as airtight as possible.

For internal use, take 1–2 tbsp. (or standard spoonfuls) as needed for benefits – or combine with vinegar and add to fresh greens or salads. Apply to unbroken skin for topical benefits, depending on the herb (see monographs).

• Double Boiler Infused Oil

Why use a double boiler? Oils can be volatile (and smoky) when overheated. Even if left unattended only briefly, an unsupervised stovetop-infused oil could reach a boil or simmer quite quickly. Not only would this ruin the final product, it could

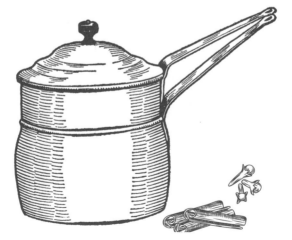

pose a fire hazard, as oils can catch fire if they become too hot.

When going this route, purchase a good oil with a high smoke point. (Be careful not to exceed the smoke point: check the oil temperature regularly with a clean meat thermometer.) Smoking oil can pose a fire hazard, of course, but it can also destroy any health properties and nutrients in the herbs.

Personal favourites for the double boiler infused oil are sunflower seed oil, avocado oil, almond oil, olive oil, jojoba and coconut oil – the latter two are wonderful for skin-nourishment salves, especially accompanied by aloe. Again, some of these have lower smoke points and will therefore require a more watchful eye to avoid · burning. You can either use a proper double boiler, or fashion a rudimentary one, which is explained in the following steps.

STEP 1 – Place a measurement of herbs in a clean stovetop pot (preferably stainless steel) and pour oil over the herbs. If using a double boiler, place the herbs and oil in the top chamber.
STEP 2 – In a separate stovetop pot (with a copper bottom), place a good level of water for a consistent boil of 1–2 hours. (If using a double boiler, add this water to the bottom chamber.)

Obviously, the higher the volume of herbs and oil you plan on infusing, the higher the volume of water should be. (As a general rule, equal parts of water and oil work well.)

STEP 3 – Place the double boiler setup on the stove and bring the water in the lower pot to a boil with the oil- and herb-filled pot set on top. Once it reaches a boil, turn down the heat slightly, to a strong simmer.

STEP 4 – Let the oil simmer for at least 1 to 2 hours. You are free to infuse it longer, if desired. If the oil changes colour, you'll know that it has begun to take on the compounds in the infusing herbs (most, but not all, oils will change colour in response to taking on herbal compounds).

STEP 5 – Once satisfied with the infusion, turn down the heat and let cool. Once cooled to a lukewarm temperature, strain the oil with a fine strainer or piece of cheesecloth into another container (you may use an empty, cleaned cooking-oil bottle; be sure to label it).

STEP 6 – Store in a cool, dry place and make sure the bottle or container is as airtight as possible. **For internal use, take 1–2 tbsp. (or standard spoonfuls) as needed for benefits – or combine with vinegar and add to fresh greens or salads. Apply to unbroken skin for topical benefits, depending on the herb (see Monographs).**

BASIC SALVE

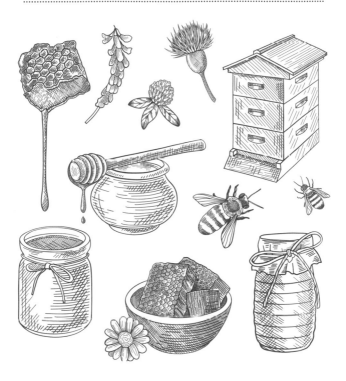

Any infused oil can be transformed into a salve
or balm with the addition of beeswax. Salves are
perfect for joint, muscle and skin issues (but not
so much for wounds) including arthritis, muscle

cramps or sunburn when rubbed into the skin, with the help of herbs like arnica, comfrey and others. Balms, of course, can be rubbed on the lips and are perfect for moistening and emollient herbs such as aloe or plantain (be sure to check out the Herbal Monographs section for more information on these).

There are differing opinions among herbalists on the perfect ratio of beeswax to oil. **I tend to take one quarter (¼) of the volume of the oil, and convert that into a solid measurement for adding into the oil (grams or solid ounces).** The same concerns about purity and sustainability of oil apply to beeswax. Make sure you're getting a pure product that is chemical- and additive-free; buying from a local beekeeper is ideal if you want to have the best quality and integrity in your salve or balm.

The steps for salve-making are simple, and preceded by the creation of either a sun-infused oil or a double boiler oil – your choice. However, if you want to make a salve in one night, or whip one up as quickly as possible, use the double boiler method and not the sun-infused one.

That said, you can still create a salve from sun-infused oil; the directions will just vary (see the following steps). In either case, make sure you have your salve jars ready before you start

– these should be shallow containers into which you'll be pouring your salves to cool. For home use, I love using very small Mason jars (or Kilner jars in the UK).

First, for creating a salve, simply follow your preferred infused-oil directions. Then:

STEP 1 – While your infused oil is still hot during the creation process (and the heat is turned off), drop in your measurement of beeswax and let it dissolve in the hot oil in your double boiler. If you are making a sun-infused oil into a salve, you can take your final product here and place it in the top chamber of your double boiler. Bring it up to a heat level that will melt the beeswax, then add your wax (again, while the heat is turned off).

STEP 2 – While still hot, stir the oil with a stainless-steel spoon to make sure the wax is fully incorporated – but only do this briefly. While the oil and beeswax mixture is still quite hot, pour into your salve jars. If you're after a particular salve 'consistency', you have the option of letting the mixture cool in the pot (you'll find out why in the next step).

STEP 3 – Once fully cooled in the jars (if you choose this option), your salves are ready. But, if you (like me) are picky about your salve's consistency, the process doesn't have to end here.

Depending on the oil and herbs you use – especially if you're using fresh herbs, which can add water to the final product – even the most well-measured oil-to-wax ratio can bring you an undesirable salve consistency. It can sometimes be on the runny side, no matter how closely you follow directions.

Checking and correcting salve consistency: To find out if the consistency meets your requirements (and correct it), test the mixture with a spoon and rub it into your fingers. Scrape some off the top of your cooled mixture (if you left it to cool in the double boiler); if it cooled in the jars, take some from there (although it may ruin that nice, smooth final 'lip balm' appearance).

My favourite way to salve consistency: there is almost always some residue from the salve in the double boiler, even if you poured it off into your jars. However, here's the advantage of simply letting it cool in the double boiler: if it's not quite the right consistency, you can just get the burner going and heat it up again.

With the jars, you'll have to scoop your salve back into the double boiler again (unless you're pretty confident of the consistency). My method will save you time and mess.

Too runny? Add more beeswax, and melt it in. **Not soft enough?** Add a bit more oil, which will dilute the final product, but still render it useful. After this, let the salve cool again in your preferred way, check the consistency again, and repeat as many times as necessary until you get the consistency you like.

Once complete, apply salve topically as needed onto unbroken skin (or superficial wounds or burns, if using a wound or burn healer like aloe or pine).

POULTICE

Using herbs topically doesn't require an elaborate recipe. Poultices are a perfect example of this; they are typically whipped up on the spot for topical use and are very effective (and safe) for non-serious superficial cuts, wounds, burns, bug bites, or anything that could be infected. They are also appropriate for other topical uses.

A poultice is basically a crushed-up mixture or plaster of herbs, preferably fresh (some of them are quite 'sensational', to say the least). Some great gentle poultice candidates are comfrey, arnica, and plantain (the last of which is popular as a rudimentary 'Spit Poultice' – see p. 160). Other 'intense' herbs like mustard seed, peppermint and even cayenne pepper or garlic have therapeutic effects as poultices, but can be too intense for some.

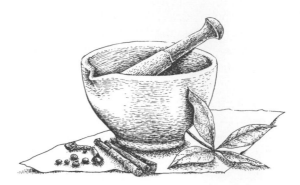

That said, if it's something you wish to try (considering the caustic cautions) your poultice could have some aloe gel or other soothing compound for the skin added to lessen uncomfortable chemical reactions. It's a fair price to pay for a proper poultice, one of the oldest and most powerful herbal preparation remedies.

STEP 1 – Gather the fresh herbs or spices you plan to use. Also gather any 'binders' or other ingredients you may wish to add to your poultice for additional effects: some use flour, corn meal (polenta), cooking oil or a bit of aloe gel to make it into a soothing paste, or to allow the poultice to stick to the skin (keep in mind skin allergens, of course – especially to flour, wheat and gluten). However, binders aren't essential.

STEP 2 – Using your preferred method, grind your herbs. You may use a culinary coffee grinder, food processor, blender or cheese grater (with herbal roots such as comfrey). Or do it the old-fashioned way, by hand with a mortar and pestle. Grind your additives or binders in with these. Regardless, make sure you use clean tools.

Fresh herbs can also be simply chopped up or finely minced with a well-sharpened chef's knife.

STEP 3 – Apply the poultice to the affected area. Keep in mind (and prepare yourself for) any chemical reaction that may occur with more caustic herbs on wounds, burns etc. (such as mint or mustard). Avoid this type of application altogether if you're uncertain of your pain tolerance.

For respiratory issues, or to ease breathing, apply poultices to the chest or neck, so they can be inhaled and open up your air passages (think of a vapour rub here). Poultices are also popular for intramuscular pain or to speed the healing of bones and ligaments without broken skin (arnica and comfrey come to mind for this). Once the desired effect is achieved, rinse away herbal matter and cleanse skin.

SYRUPS

The herbal cough syrup has a long place and history in the herbalism world – and obviously a sweet spot, too. One of the most favoured (and flavoured) vehicles for respiratory herbs, syrups can also be made for enjoyment first and natural healing second – not just for soothing coughs or sore throats, but also for flavouring teas, cocktails and foods.

The best part? You're already more than halfway to a syrup when you create a strong

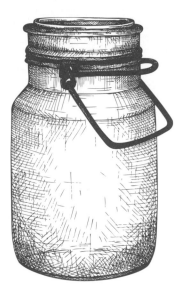

infusion or decoction. The rest is easy. I've worked with many different ratios and have done a lot of eyeballing over the years when making my syrups, which happen to be one of my favourite preparations. One part honey to two parts water for syrup has generally worked out for me, although three parts water has worked as well. However, much like other herbal preparations (I'm thinking of herbal salves here), I adjust herbal syrups for consistency at the very end.

STEP 1 – Refer to the sections above on either infusions or decoctions to get your herbal syrup going – your choice will depend on the herb (or herbs) you wish to use.

The syrup-making process begins when the herbs are fully filtered or strained out of the final infusion or decoction product and placed back into a large enough stovetop pot (preferably with a copper bottom) and ready to reheat on the stove.

STEP 2 – Measure your honey (using a roughly 1:2 honey to water ratio) and add to the stovetop pot. Bring all of this to a boil. Once a boil is reached, turn it down to medium-low, or a strong but low simmer.

STEP 3 – Simmering time for your syrup can vary, but usually lasts 1 hour, sometimes up to 2 hours (depending, of course, on the volume of syrup you are making). Either way, if you're making a syrup, it is something to stick around for and watch, to make sure it does not overboil.

As it simmers, you can also check the consistency of your syrup with a stainless-steel spoon (wait for it to cool and give it a taste for mouthfeel, thickness, etc.). Once it reaches your desired consistency, it is finished – it could be a more watery or runny syrup, or thicker in consistency, your choice, though you obviously don't want a syrup that's *too* runny.

You also have the option of boiling the mixture all the way down for the thickest syrup possible. You'll know the mixture cannot be boiled down any thicker when the syrup begins to actively 'foam', rising up to the edge of the stovetop pot. At this point, be sure to turn off the heat and remove it from the burner immediately, before it overflows. (This is why it's wise to stay close and keep an eye on your syrup.)

STEP 4 – Let the syrup cool down completely. Store in clean jars or bottles that close tightly, and keep it refrigerated. Unlike pure honey, herbal syrups are not shelf-stable, as they may contain water harbouring microbes (usually mould) that may grow on the top layer of your syrup.

Use your syrups within 6 to 12 months. **Take 1–2 tbsp. (or standard spoonfuls) as needed**

for benefits (first, be sure to check 'Warnings Before Use' with any herb you make syrup from in this book). As you use them, you may start to notice their flavour waning, so use them quickly – it's a sign that their wellness benefits could be slipping away too. Herbs in this book that make pleasant-tasting syrups are lemon balm, angelica, white pine, sumac and even agrimony. These herbal syrups can also improve the flavour of less palatable remedies, such as valerian root or lion's mane.

VINEGARS AND SHRUBS

In the same vein as syrups, vinegars and preparations made with them hold a special place in the herbal world (and in my heart). No medium is better at extracting and preserving vitamins and minerals – and much can be done to make them flavourful, enjoyable and unique, in addition to remedial.

Herbs known to be nutrient dense, like stinging nettle, lion's mane and other medicinal mushrooms (shiitake, reishi etc.) are fantastic candidates for herbal vinegars. Obviously, your favourite culinary seasoning herbs – garlic, rosemary, sage and the like – can make for intriguing vinegars for both food and wellness use. Sour or 'piney' flavoured herbs (juniper, pine, rhubarb or sumac) can have the best brought out in them flavour-wise with the help of a simple, light vinegar – and their properties are preserved too.

Opt for vinegars that are pure, light and have no other ingredients, such as white vinegar or rice vinegar (avoid balsamic or flavoured vinegar). Apple cider vinegar is one of my favourites if you

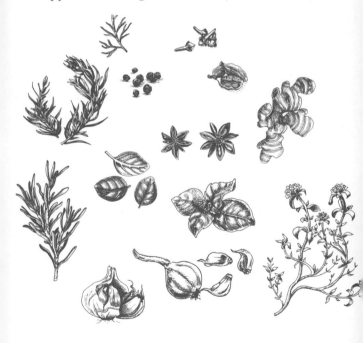

want to add a touch of fermentation, and you get all the health benefits of ACV mixed into your creation, too.

Vinegars are straightforward preparations. I personally do not follow a ratio for creating a herbal vinegar. I simply fill up the entire container I plan to use with my preferred herbs.

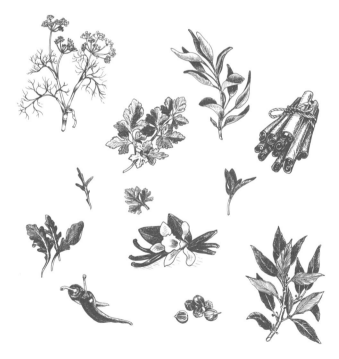

SIMPLE VINEGAR

STEP 1 – Take a clean, closeable container (a Mason/Kilner jar works well) and fill it with a herb or combination of herbs.

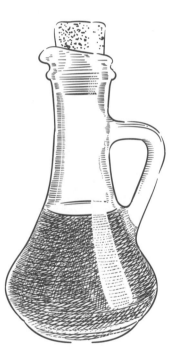

STEP 2 – Cover the herbs with the vinegar of your choice and seal it tightly. Keep in mind: if

you're using steel or any type of metal lid, place a section of greaseproof paper, baking parchment or even newspaper in between the mouth of the jar and the lid. This protects the metal from being oxidized by the vinegar, which can cause the lid to rust and foul up your vinegar.

STEP 3 – Shake the jar vigorously when closed, then refrigerate for a week to infuse. If you're using apple cider vinegar and would like a touch of fermentation in the mix (not much – only a subtle raise in probiotic acetic acid bacteria), leave it to infuse at room temperature for 24 hours, then refrigerate.

STEP 4 – Over the course of the week, whenever you think of it, give the jar a shake. This will help release more herbal compounds and flavours (and it's a nice bicep workout, honestly).

STEP 5 – After the week is over, put the vinegar through a fine strainer to remove all herbal matter. Bottle the final product in a glass jar or bottle. Don't forget to create a barrier between the mouths of your containers and any metal lids to prevent oxidation and spoilage.

Store your vinegar in the fridge. For short periods of time, it can be kept at room temperature in a dark, dry place. I recommend using the vinegar within 6 to 12 months.

Take 1–2 tbsp. (or standard spoonfuls) of vinegar

internally as needed, or mix into greens or salads.
(First, be sure to check 'Warnings Before Use' with
any herb you make vinegar from in this book.)

TINCTURES, EXTRACTS AND BITTERS

Herbalists consider tinctures (alcohol-preserved
preparations of herbs) the ultimate herbal
creation, and one of the best ways to store and
use herbs effectively over the long term. Although
they may sound intimidating, they are probably
the easiest preparations to make.

Then there are the close relatives of the
tincture: bitters. These tend to focus more on
promoting digestion (as an aperitif or digestif)
and showcasing a flavour or flavour combo
(though not always), and they take a little extra
craftsmanship to make...though not much.
Tinctures, on the other hand, usually don't taste
very good (I'm being honest here). Some herbs,
when simply extracted, are very tasty (such as
agrimony, hops or sumac). Tinctures also steep (or
'macerate') much longer than bitters, which are
made overnight.

**Another difference between tinctures and
bitters: with the former, you'll want the highest
proof possible for optimal extraction of herbal
compounds.** In these instances, a good grade

Everclear or vodka tends to be favourable (it should be a clear alcohol). With bitters, however, you can use other types of liquor, even flavoured or non-clear types such as gin, rum, whiskey, tequila or bourbon.

For the best tincture-making ratios, and creating high-quality extractions and products, I can't recommend Richo Cech's *Making Plant*

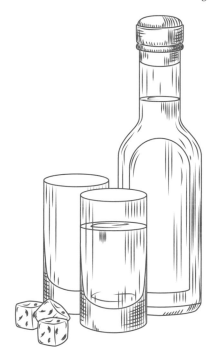

Medicine enough to get those skills fine-tuned. The book discusses all the possible types of compounds in herbs, the best ways to extract them, and the best ratio of alcohol to water.

For quick creations that will still have good benefits for home use and preserve your herbs for upwards of 10 years, however, this simple recipe will be more than adequate.

For any of these tinctures, take as little as 15-30 drops as needed or per day, or 1-2 dropperfuls per day or per setting for healing benefits. **Make sure to educate yourself about the potential side effects, warnings, or interactions noted under each herbal monograph.**

For digestive bitters, take a few drops (on tongue or in drinkable glass of water) before or after meals to boost digestion.

BASIC TINCTURE OR EXTRACT

STEP 1 – Make sure your herb is well processed, meaning it is dried all the way down, leaves removed from stems, or better yet ground down or minced into a powder or chopped as finely as possible. This will assist in extracting all the right compounds into your tincture.

Tough roots, seeds or nuts may require additional processing with a grinder or food

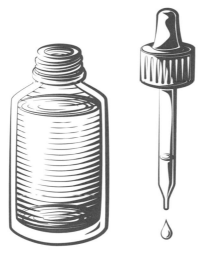

processor. You can use herbs of all kinds in their fresh form for tinctures.

STEP 2 – Place the herb in a clean Mason/Kilner jar or other container that is food safe and airtight. Pour your high-proof alcohol over the herbal matter until it's substantially submerged, but not so much that there is significantly more alcohol than herbal matter. (I find that roughly 1 part herbal matter to 1.5–2 parts alcohol works well.)

If you are tincturing dry herbal matter, add a splash of water. Many herbs have a diversity of compounds, some extracted in alcohol and some in water (either alcohol or water soluble) so a little extra water to make up for the loss of an herb's natural water weight helps. Alcohol does contain some water to help with cold water extraction of these compounds, too.

STEP 3 – Store the jar in a cool, dark place for one month. Whenever you think of it, give it a good shake. This can help loosen compounds for infusion and extraction.

STEP 4 – After a month, put the tincture through a fine strainer or cheesecloth into a separate clean container. Store it in a dark place, preferably in dark amber glass containers (blue or green work well too). I recommend using dropper bottles for tinctures and keeping them there when the tincture is complete. This makes them easy to use and readily available, taking drops or droppers here and there at a time.

BITTERS RECIPES

Most bitters are made with a focus on digestion. They can incorporate digestion-forward herbs like lemon balm, angelica, hops and culinary classics like mint, fennel or ginger.

STEP 1 – Make sure your herb is well processed, meaning it is dried all the way down, leaves removed from stems, or better yet ground down or minced into a powder or chopped as finely as possible. This will assist in extracting all the right compounds into your bitters.

Tough roots, seeds or nuts may require additional processing with a grinder or food processor. You can use herbs of all kinds in their fresh form for tinctures and bitters. If you're making bitters with multiple herbs, make sure you choose herbs that will taste good together and that, to an extent, share similar health properties too. Many people add strongly flavoured foods, spices and seasonings to bitters to enhance their flavour profile: orange zest, lemon juice, fruits, star anise or even smoked salts.

STEP 2 – Place all the ingredients in a clean Mason/Kilner jar or other container that is food safe and airtight. Pour alcohol over the ingredients until they are substantially submerged.

STEP 3 – Store the jar in a cool, dark place overnight. Give it a good shake a few times when you remember it.

STEP 4 – The next day, put the bitters concoction through a fine strainer or cheesecloth into a separate clean container. Store your bitters in a dark place, preferably in dark amber glass containers (blue or green work well too).

Just like with tinctures, I recommend using dropper bottles with bitters and keeping them there when the tincture is complete. This makes them easy to use when you need them, taking drops or droppers here and there at a time, such as an aperitif or digestif before and after meals.

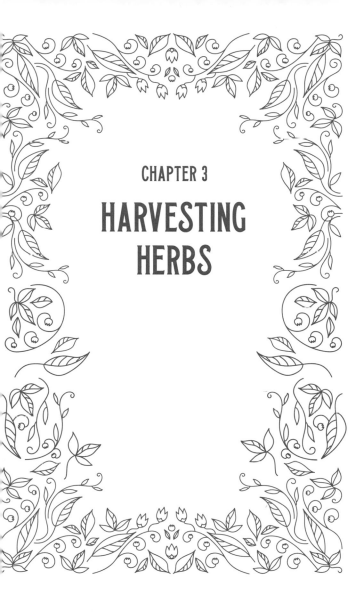

CHAPTER 3
HARVESTING HERBS

Herb and supplement companies exist to meet your herbal healing needs: loose leaf teas, teabags, sifted spices, tinctures, extracts, syrups…the list goes on. Still, pretty much every acolyte reaches a point where they wish to explore sourcing their own, often in addition to or for the purpose of making their own products. Harvesting herbs for personal use or self-care, also called 'wildcrafting', can be one of the greatest delights for the budding or expert herbalist. It can help you feel more in control of your health, wellness, vitality and nutrition.

You can wildcraft your own herbal remedies and personal medicines, or you can take things a step further and grow your own cultivars.

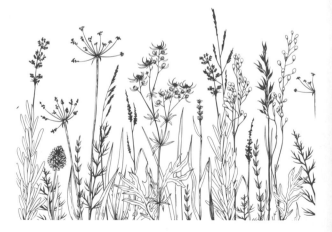

(You may also wish to become the steward of a local weed patch or other natural area.) While harvesting herbs may seem like a straightforward and intuitive process, there are more than a few things that first-time herb harvesters should know before they get started. In this section, you will find basic guidance and how-to's for the most common category of herbal parts.

❧ Guidance on harvesting herbs in urban areas

Live in the city and wonder if harvesting herbs is possible for you? The answer is yes, it's absolutely possible – but you must be mindful of waste sites, contamination and pollution. Obviously, many urbanites grow gardens or plots without a hitch, picking and harvesting herbal remedies that are clean, pure and without contamination from chemicals in the soil or air. These, in the end, are perfectly safe for consumption. However, it does require one to be mindful of the plot and placement of one's garden area. Strategy in where you plant is very important.

It's best to grow and nurture your herbs away from roads, especially well-travelled ones where smog and pollution could settle on your plants (and thus into your body when you consume them). When growing your own herbs, be mindful of where your home (if planting in the ground) is located. Is it in a recent waste site? Did there used to be a home there? Is it downhill from a road or train track? You're safer not growing into the ground directly, and better off sourcing your own potting soil and cultivating herbs in raised beds far above the ground and away from contamination. If you are not sure about the safety of the site, you can test the soil for heavy metals, radioactive materials, and contaminants before you begin.

If you're not growing your own herbs, you might be surprised at the number of wild plant varieties in your city or neighbourhood that have medicinal qualities – such as stinging nettle, sumac and pine. Regardless, the above considerations apply to wild herbs you find in the city too. Avoid harvesting from plants near roads or downhill from suspicious chemical- or pollution-laden areas. If harvesting from a public park, it's wise to get in touch with the authorities to find out if they spray certain areas (and to check whether it is acceptable to harvest herbs from the park to begin with). Runoff from high spray areas – like lawns, golf courses etc. – are something to consider too.

Be especially wary of thick clumps of annual herbs growing near waste sites in cities. While these may look absolutely tantalizing because of

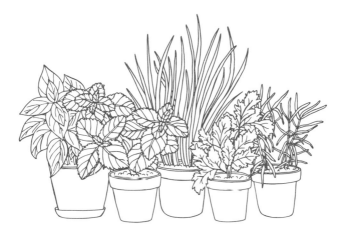

the sheer volume growing in one place (this is especially common with herbs like the European species of stinging nettle), these 'clumps' are often evidence of a high accumulation of harmful chemicals or heavy metals. You will want to avoid harvesting from these, as it's likely these herbs are acting as 'bio-accumulators' sucking up chemicals from the earth, which you will then consume.

✿ Guidance on harvesting herbs in rural areas

If you live near a pristine natural area, such as a national or state park (or wildlife refuge), it may feel like the world is your oyster when it comes to herb harvesting. And that may be true. You're

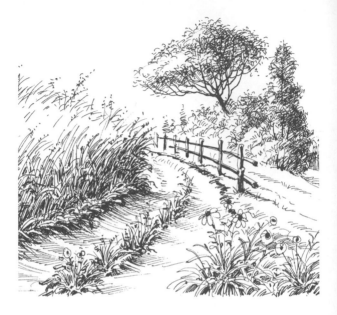

more likely to find a wide variety of healing herbs in the wild, as well as mushroom healers like lion's mane in untouched wilderness. But that's not to say there won't be barriers to wildcrafting in rural areas.

The same rules apply to the country, especially if you live near agricultural areas. Make sure to consider not only chemical runoff or pollution from roads or waste sites into wild areas you may be harvesting from, but also look out for the runoff from farm fields and ditches. These can pose health hazards through the very plants you wish to pick for the purpose of healing.

If you have a lot of natural wilderness at your disposal – such as mountains, desert, forest, prairie or wetlands – it's also wise to make sure that the harvesting of any herb in these areas is *allowable*. Even without signs posted, walking off-trail in a public park or wildlife refuge could damage plant species or other wildlife. If it's not your own property but is a public area, always enquire with the government or local body managing the area if foot traffic is admissible. Do not trespass onto private property in search of herbal remedies without obtaining the owner's express permission.

❦ Guidance on harvesting herbs respectfully, sustainably and ethically

Especially when harvesting herbs from the wild, be mindful of how much you are harvesting; this can apply when harvesting herbs in your own garden, too. Clearly, pulling out or depleting your plot will mean fewer herbs and a less vibrant patch in the future. The same goes for wild herbs. Ask yourself how much of the herb you really need. Will others (including animals and other

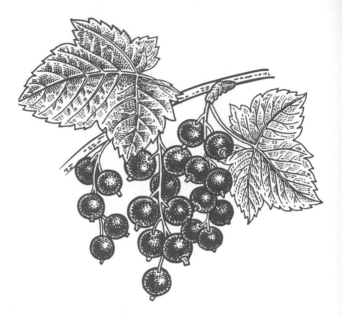

wildlife) be depending on or using the herbs growing here too?

While it can be tempting to harvest all the herbs you find (especially when finding a more elusive herb, and especially when you are harvesting its roots), good ethics among herbalists insist that you take only what you need – and be mindful of the wild population to ensure that it can continue to be just that: a wild, self-sustaining population that will thrive and produce herbal remedies for years to come. If overharvested or stressed, you put the source of your very herbal health and wellness at risk – not just the wellbeing of the plant population.

The health and welfare of a wild stand of herbs is something to take into consideration if you want to wildcraft your home remedies in the most respectful way. Avoid overharvesting from any population, small or large. Be particularly careful of overharvesting from a single plant: its seeds, flowers, leaves, aerial parts or fruiting parts especially, which plants need to both feed themselves and reproduce. When picking your remedies from a population, try to spread out what you take from the population instead of concentrating on one particular area.

A good hard-and-fast rule is to only take up to one third of the available harvestable parts or plants (if harvesting roots) from a population – and only take up to one third of the available seeds, flowers, berries or fruit from a single plant at a time, or from that population. If harvesting the full one third, avoid harvesting from that population or patch for a while to give it time to recover and replenish.

Herbalists are often drawn to working with plants knowing full well they're creating relationships with living things – and living things deserve respect. Harvesting respectfully, in the work and practice of many herbalists, is integral to building a relationship with any plant or remedy.

In the beliefs of some, this relationship can even ensure or enhance the potency of the preparations you make with them. In the spirit of ancient herbalist practices that involve magick or spiritualism too, some may even turn to certain traditions for honouring or thanking plants that they harvest from – leaving gifts, offerings or tokens with the plants as a 'thank you' or respectful trade to be able to experience their medicines. Herbalists of many backgrounds have their own rituals around this, based on ancestry or culture, or they may develop personal rituals.

One of my favourite offerings (when harvesting seeds, fruits or berries) is to take a pinch of the berries, seeds, fruits or even fruiting bodies (in the case of wild mushrooms) of whatever I'm harvesting and spread them to new areas – unless they are more invasively inclined. My trade is to aid them in their reproduction process, helping them strengthen or expand their population, and also to ensure there is more life for them – and more herbal remedies for me and others – for years to come as part of our symbiotic herbalist-herb relationship. If you are seeking an equitable ritual, this one has a spiritual and logical basis.

❧ Harvesting herbal 'aerial parts' (leaves, stems, whole herb etc.)

Most herbs you'll harvest and work with will be made up of 'aerial parts' – the above-ground portion of the plant, usually leaves and stems of a tender nature (such as agrimony, mugwort, plantain or lemon balm). In some cases, it means leaves only, especially if the herbal twigs and branches are of a tougher nature – such as with pine needles, the 'leaves' of the pine tree,

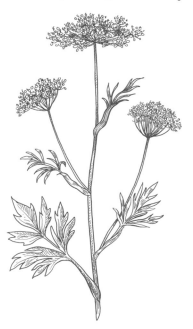

which are harvested while leaving the tougher twigs behind (though that doesn't necessarily mean these tougher parts don't have healing properties too).

If harvesting the entire aerial part of a plant (the whole herb, down to the root), use plant cutters or a strong knife to cut the main stem of the herb right down and close to the ground. Remove the whole herb, and use as directed in your preparation. If only leaves are to be used (as in the case of pine), harvest these individually from the plant by hand without cutting out the entire plant – which would be a challenge with a plant like pine, anyway.

✿ Harvesting herbal flowers

If the herb in question is a tender annual or perennial, harvesting flowers tends to be a breeze (and this is usually the case for the feature flower remedies in this book, arnica and hops). You can gently remove blossoms from stems with your thumb and forefinger, taking care to leave around two-thirds of the flowers or blossoms so that the herb you are harvesting from can still reproduce with its seeds.

If it is a tougher-stemmed plant, scissors or gardening snips can be helpful for removing flowers – roses from rose bushes are a good example. Hops flowers (the cones or 'strobiles' considered a flowering part of the vine) can have a tougher nature in some cases, and have an easier time being harvested with a sharper tool. Some herbalists favour putting their flowers in a shallow wicker or reed basket, being careful to layer blossoms only one layer deep and using the basket to hold the flowers as they air dry naturally.

❦ Harvesting herbal seeds

Harvesting seeds is very similar in spirit to harvesting herbal flowers. In most cases they

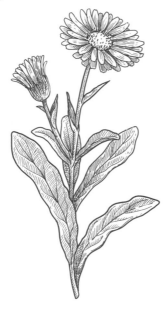

can be easily removed by hand, and with a simple plucking of your fingers, seed by seed into a container. Herbs with monographs in this book – like stinging nettle, angelica and milk thistle – have harvestable seeds. Some herbalists prefer to cut whole flowers or drupes, and then hang them to dry, just like herbal aerial parts; removing the seeds may be easier when they are dried. This is often the way milk thistle seeds are harvested, dried and stored for later use or herbal

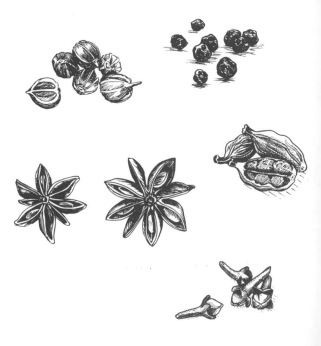

preparation (see p. 146 for harvesting method). That said, drying the seeds isn't necessary, unless you would like to store them for the long term in your cabinet or apothecary. Otherwise, if you have the patience, freshly harvested seeds have amazing potency compared to dried, including stronger aromatic compounds, oils and phytochemicals (especially with fragrant remedies, like angelica). The only downside: the harvesting of fresh seeds takes longer. In the case of harvesting dry seeds, removing the flower to dry the seeds can be easier using a sharp knife, scissors, or plant cutter rather than just your hands.

🌿 Harvesting herbal berries or fruits

You'll find that harvesting herbal berries and fruits has a lot in common with seeds, although it's a much easier process thanks to the larger average size of these plant parts. This book's exemplary berry remedy, sumac, grows in clusters, or 'drupes', that are simple to process and create with, and without having to remove all berries to be effective. With other herbal fruits, however – such as elderberry or hawthorn (not explored in this book) – berries tend to be easier to remove from their stems or drupes, and it is preferred to use them that way. Just as in seeds, tougher drupes to remove (such as sumac) may be easier

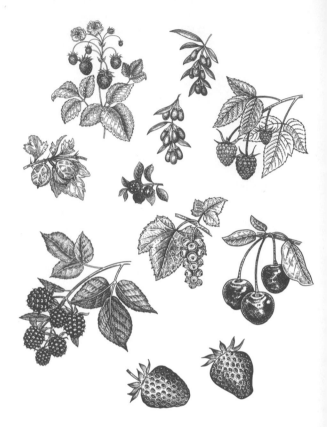

and more convenient with the help of a sharp tool. In more tender plants, fruits or berries can be easily removed and picked with one's fingers. After harvesting, it is often recommended to use most fruits and berries right away; otherwise, dry them (if possible), though this may sap some berries of their medicinal qualities. Because of their combined sugar and water content, fresh herbal fruit or berry remedies simply don't have much of a shelf life, and are best preserved in syrups, vinegars or tinctures.

℘ Harvesting herbal roots

Herbal roots rank among the most powerful remedies you can harvest, preserve and use for self-care and healing. In exchange for their incredible benefits and potency, they may involve the most work to extract – or more accurately, to exhume (dig up). One of this book's feature root remedies, comfrey, will almost certainly require a shovel or spade; it has a long taproot that delves deep into the ground. Valerian is a similar root remedy that grows deep – and, as a rule, the larger the root is, the more time and digging it will take to pull up.

Garlic, on the other hand, tends to be a shallow cultivated grower. Still, many growers harvest these bulbs with the aid of a shovel or, at the very least, a hand spade. In some cases, the earth is soft enough to pull these combination pot-herb/vegetables from the ground with little to no effort. Upon removal, you will want to remove by hand

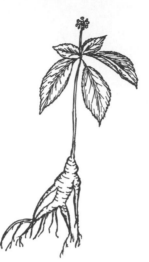

any clumped dirt from herbal roots, or rinse or scrub it away before using it fresh in preparations or drying it for storage. With all root remedies, the best time to harvest is in the autumn or early winter, when plants send the most energy to their underground systems. This means that the root is more likely to have plentiful compounds for health, healing and nutritive purposes too. Some herbalists choose very early spring as their second choice time for harvesting herbal roots.

❧ Harvesting mushroom fruiting bodies

Mushrooms are becoming popular herbal remedies in a lot of circles. As such, it's important to know how to properly harvest these medicinal treasures. This book's resident fungal healer, lion's mane, is only one example among many well-reputed, wellness-boosting mushrooms including cordyceps, reishi, maitake, chaga, shiitake and more that unfortunately could not be fully explored in this book. Though obviously these are not plant remedies, they can be compared to plants in that the fruiting body (the most easily and commonly used medicinal part) is much like the fungi's 'flower'.

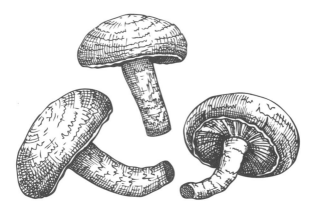

With some delicacy and finesse, harvesting tender mushroom fruiting bodies (e.g. lion's mane, maitake, shiitake, portobello, etc.) takes only your thumb and forefinger. Regardless of the species, find where the tender 'stem' of the fruiting body emerges from the tree bark, wood chips, or other medium. Pinch tightly and pull away to remove.

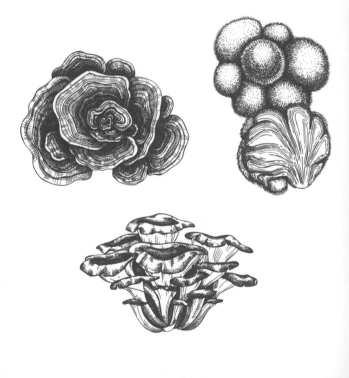

With tougher mushroom fruiting bodies (such as reishi, but especially for chaga mushroom), you may need a strong knife or hatchet to harvest in the same way: removing the fruiting body from the tree at its base, but with more sustained effort.

A note on wildcrafting mushrooms: be sure to introduce yourself to wild healing mushroom

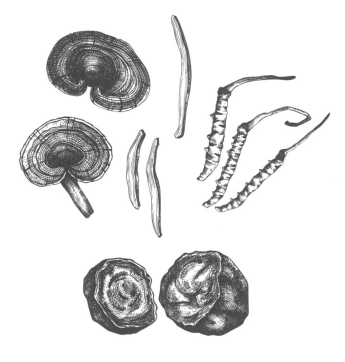

remedies with the help of a local guide or expert before wildcrafting them on your own. There are far too many poisonous lookalikes, and mushroom harvesting can end badly – even in death – due to naiveté. It is essential that you learn or are guided by failsafe identification first.

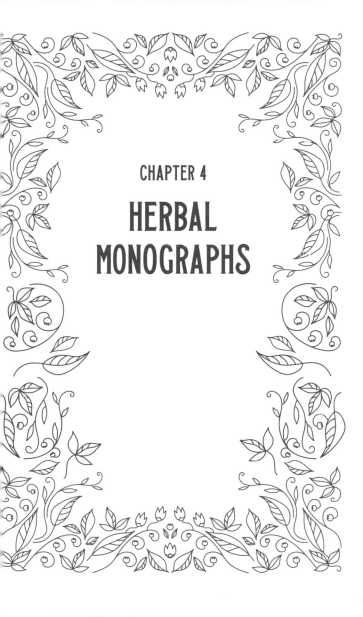

CHAPTER 4

HERBAL MONOGRAPHS

Explore these 16 herbs that I (and other herbalists) have found so much joy working with on a culinary level, a self-healing level, or both. I couldn't possibly fit everything there is to know and every possible healing benefit into this book, so I hope readers are satisfied with these introductions – helped along (hopefully) by sharing my personal experiences with them as briefly and as helpfully as I can.

A quick, handy guide to using this section as an easy reference: In each herbal monograph, you will find recommendations of the parts to use and the best preparations to use with each of these plants or mushrooms. Look at the 'Parts Used' section under each herb, and cross-reference with the 'Harvesting Herbs' chapter, depending on which part of the remedy you are harvesting, to find basic instructions. Look at the 'Best Preparations' section under each entry, and cross-reference with the 'Basic Herbal Preparations' chapter to find instructions on how to make a basic remedy (or more than one type of remedy) of said herb or mushroom.

Keep the possibility of contact or food allergies to any of these herbs in mind when using them internally. I'd recommend using a small patch or skin test beforehand, to see what happens first. If your skin becomes inflamed, I would avoid using the herb altogether because yes, allergies and severe reactions are possible. If at any point, internal use of an herb is causing nausea, vomiting, confusion, stomach upset or other symptoms of bad food reaction, discontinue its use immediately.

Included under each profile entry are some interesting and more specialized (to the plant) preparations or recipes contributed by herbalists, chefs and other experts I know and look up to. Some of my own are included in the mix. While I don't claim strong ownership over any of my herbal recipes, some of these preparations are the herbalist's or specialist's own iterations of preparations that are as old as humanity – while others are branded as their own inventions, or methods they have taken pride in developing. Keep this in mind and with respect as you create.

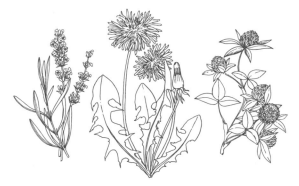

❦ Glossary of herbalism terms

The following terms will be shown under each herbal profile, designating a general overview of the purported health benefits of each herb. These terms are often used by herbalists. Reference this section to get acquainted with what each herb can do.

ADAPTOGEN – May help the body 'adapt' to stress, inflammation, ageing and disease (somewhat synonymous with immune-boosting or tonic).

ALTERATIVE – May help support detoxifying functions of the body through kidneys and liver, 'blood cleanser'.

ANALGESIC – May help reduce mild pain. (Also called 'Anodyne'.)

ANTI-ALLERGIC – May help support the body when dealing with allergies.

ANTIBACTERIAL – May help support the body when dealing with bacterial infection.

ANTIBIOTIC – May help support the body when dealing with infection from bacteria, fungi, protozoa or other living microorganisms by making the bodily environment unlivable temporarily.

ANTI-DIABETIC – May help the body better regulate blood sugars.

ANTI-DIARRHOEAL – May help support symptoms of diarrhoea.

ANTIFUNGAL – May help support the body when dealing with fungal infections or overgrowth.

ANTIHISTAMINE – May help the body reduce a mild histamine or allergic response (e.g. pet dander, seasonal allergens, pollen etc.)

ANTI-INFLAMMATORY – May help soothe or fight inflammation.

ANTI-MICROBIAL – May help the body expel or destroy any foreign microbes or pathogens (bacteria, viruses etc.)

ANTI-PARASITIC – May help support the body in expelling parasites.

ANTISEPTIC – When used topically or on surfaces, may help partially or completely destroy pathogens that could be harmful or cause infection (bacteria, viruses etc.)

ANTI-SPASMODIC – May help the body reduce muscle contractions and spasms, e.g. cramping.

ANTI-VIRAL – May help support the body when dealing with viruses or viral infections.

ASTRINGENT – Dries, tightens, 'contracts' and tonifies on contact or after consumption of

either tissues or skin (think of the actions of a 'skin toner' versus emollient action). Also denotes anti-diarrhoeal digestive support.

CARDIOTONIC – Supports cardiovascular health (blood vessels, blood pressure, arterial walls etc.)

CARMINATIVE – May relieve gas and flatulence.

DECONGESTANT – May help the body relieve upper respiratory congestion.

DEMULCENT – Similar to emollient but specifically effective against inflammation (may also denote laxative action).

DIAPHORETIC – May help the body break a fever, typically administered in the form of a hot tea, infusion or decoction.

DISCUTIENT – May help disperse 'stuck' tissue or matter in the body; usually applies to blood clots or bruising.

DIGESTIVE BITTER – May promote digestion by stimulating release of peptides, bile flow, or reintroducing natural digestive enzymes.

DIURETIC – May help promote urination, which may support detoxification, liver health, kidney health, purify the body's lymphatic system and reduce gall or kidney stones.

EMMENAGOGUE – May help the body trigger the

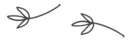

end of the menstruation cycle (bring on period – a side effect of phytoestrogen).

EMOLLIENT – For topical herbs, helps soften and moisten skin (versus astringent action). May also denote some laxative action.

EXPECTORANT – May help the upper respiratory tract (lungs, sinuses, mouth, throat etc.) produce and/or move phlegm to aid in fighting an infection or dealing with upper respiratory symptoms.

FEBRIFUGE – May help cool or reduce a fever.

GALACTAGOGUE – May help stimulate lactation in women while pregnant (side effect of phytoestrogen).

HEPATOPROTECTIVE – May help protect the liver from acute damage, such as from poisonous plants or fungi, chemicals, medications, alcohol, toxins etc.

HYPOTENSIVE – May help support the body in naturally lowering blood pressure.

IMMUNOMODULATOR – May help the immune system balance itself, which can be helpful for autoimmune issues.

IMMUNOSTIMULANT – May acutely trigger an aggressive immune response from the immune system to fight an infection or other threat.

MUCILAGINOUS – Produces or secretes plant mucilage that has soothing emollient, expectorant, demulcent or laxative action.

NERVINE – Helps support the nervous system, especially with anxiety or depression (nerve tonic; may have sedative properties).

NEUROPROTECTIVE – May help support the brain, nervous system and neurons against ageing, inflammation, neurological diseases or other symptoms and issues.

NOOTROPIC – May help enhance mental energy, cognitive function, learning, memory and other brain functions.

PHYTOESTROGEN – Mimics human estrogen in the body and can thus activate estrogen receptors, which when purposeful may have benefits for health (for both men and women, depending).

RUBEFACIENT – May increase redness or inflammation in the skin, or bring blood flow to a specific area.

SEDATIVE – May have a soothing effect on the nervous system, helping relieve stress, anxiety or sleep issues (also called narcotic, soporific, hypnotic).

STYPTIC – When used topically, may help reduce

or stop blood flow in wounds until one can find first aid or professional wound care.

TISSUE REGENERATOR – May support or enhance the body's ability to grow new tissue, bone, tendon and muscle in a certain rate or timeframe.

TONIC – Full of vitamins, minerals, antioxidants and/or phytochemicals that, when consumed daily, boost overall health in some way (or many ways), or may boost immune system.

TUSSIVE – May help relieve cough symptoms.

AGRIMONY (*Agrimonia eupatoria*, other species)

ENERGETICS: *Cool and Dry*
FLAVOUR: *Sour, Slightly Sweet*
PARTS USED: *Aerial (flowers, leaves, tender stems)*
BEST PREPARATIONS: *Tincture, Extract or Bitters. Also Tea or Infusion, Poultice, Vinegar or Shrub; Tincture, Extract or Bitters*
PROPERTIES:
Anti-allergic
Astringent
Febrifuge
Hepatoprotective
Styptic

Agrimony is one of those herbs for which I have personal testimony to its marvels, which quickly vaulted it to the top of my favourites list throughout both my training and personal use. It is not an herb you will find in the 'classic' books, or talked about too much in introductory herbal reference guides. For more about this

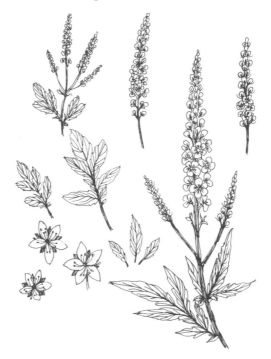

sidelined European native that has harmoniously naturalized to North America, I highly recommend herbalist Matthew Wood's book *The Book of Herbal Wisdom* (and about its close and similar relative, cinquefoil, as well); he has the same to say about agrimony's lack of fame – which is truly remarkable, considering its wonders.

I like to call certain herbs 'edge walkers' if they prefer to grow where forests start to mingle with grasslands, prairie or other more open environments. That is precisely where I first found agrimony myself (there are other species besides *Agrimonia eupatoria* that have similar uses and growing habits in the wild too). My first encounter with agrimony was delight in recognizing it in the wilds and tincturing it (the best way to use it) immediately. My expectations around the herb, and using it often or noticing powerful effects, were quite low. I was simply interested in collecting it at first – until it completely shattered my expectations.

The tinctured aerial parts of agrimony (less so a hot tea or infusion) have an aroma much like peach, apricot or strawberry: faintly fruity and little sour. I fell in love with its flavour first, which shines brightest in tincture form. A few drops add pleasant subtle flavours to fruity or citrusy drinks. On a whim, knowing it supports the liver, I happened to add a few drops to some juice while my fiancé at the time was dealing with an allergic reaction and itchiness. Its soothing effects were so immediate, I couldn't believe it, and neither could he. (Disclaimer: this benefit from agrimony is just a personal experience. It is highly possible that, based on your constitution, or differences from preparation to preparation, you will have a different experience.)

For the already seasoned herbalist or herbal practitioner, agrimony has a lot of similarity to peach leaf for the liver, inflammation and allergies – peach being another herbal remedy that I love, but that did not make it into this book. Of note, agrimony can also be a topical remedy for healing wounds and stopping bleeding until one can find first aid or professional wound care. It has strong lore and background in homeopathic healing, where it was used as a heart and blood tonic, gallbladder support, liver support and for digestive or diabetic issues that other herbalists have had their own experiences with.

WARNINGS BEFORE USE: No major considerations, though avoid consuming large quantities of the plant in one sitting (this could only be done intentionally, and would probably be an unpleasant process; it is not likely to happen by accident). Because it's high in the astringent plant compound known as tannins, it could cause some gastric upset if this is done.

Ear Ring #2 | Trilby Sedlacek, Green Angels Herbs & Healing Arts – Cedar Rapids, Iowa

Agrimony could be considered a very 'clinical' herb, so I thought this recipe 'formula' (using agrimony tincture) provided by a clinical herbalist would be a perfect pairing. Agrimony is often used as a gentle support for major issues relating to the liver or gallbladder – but also, in homeopathic tradition, for tinnitus (also called ringing in the ears). Some herbalists connect tinnitus to the cardiovascular system and blood flow, for which agrimony is considered to be a homeopathic remedy.

For beginning herbalists with ambitions to consult others for health and healing, clinical herbalist Sedlacek – registered with the American Herbalists Guild – provides this tincture formula for support with ear ringing symptoms of tinnitus. It's a fantastic example of an advanced formulation many clinical herbalists get into for creating personalized remedies for people, and which can help give beginner herbalists a taste of formulating. (Warning: Look up side effects and interactions, or speak with your doctor about these, agrimony and any other herbs you plan to take regularly.)

INGREDIENTS:
Agrimony tincture (30ml)
Bee balm tincture (100ml)
Fresh lobelia vinegar (30ml)
Ginkgo biloba tincture (60ml)
Vinca minor tincture (60ml)
Gotu kola tincture (60ml)

Directions: Take 15-20 drops in a small amount of water 2-4 times per day. If tinnitus improves, discontinue.

Says Sedlacek: 'Frequently, I add Flower essences to my formulas. This one I've added Agrimony, Pear flower or Rescue Remedy, approx. 4 drops for 60ml bottle.'

ALOE VERA (Aloe vera barbadensis)

ENERGETICS: *Cool and Damp*
FLAVOUR: *Subtly Bitter*
PARTS USED: *Latex-Free Inner Leaf Juice (internal or topical), Inner Leaf Gel or Latex (topical only)*
BEST PREPARATIONS: *Infused Oil (gel), Basic Salve (gel); Cold Tea or Cold Infusion (latex-free juice only*

if internally taken) for Compress or Wash
PROPERTIES:
Anti-diabetic (internal)
Anti-inflammatory
Demulcent
Emollient
Mucilaginous

Aloe vera is ubiquitous. And yet we take it for granted so much – I definitely have, even during my herbalism studies. Look at shampoo or other haircare or skincare product labels, and you're more likely than not to find aloe right there, listed next to other ingredients like shea butter, jojoba oil and others. Its inner mucilaginous gel is amazing at moisturizing and softening both hair and skin, and can help soothe the pain and inflammation of sunburn or first-degree burns (but is not ideal for deeper burns or wounds). While products can be made from it (see the Herbal Preparations sections indicated above), many will say that it's most beneficial when the plain inner gel is used right away.

I was also delighted to discover that when aloe's inner gel is strained into a juice – carefully processed to remove any leaf membranes and gel, which can be extremely laxative internally – it can be combined with water or other fruit juices as

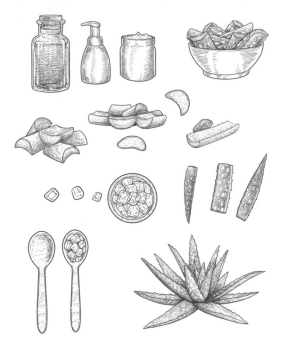

a digestive aid and to help regulate blood sugars after or between meals. As functional nutrition, aloe juice (properly sourced or made) can be a supportive remedy for those with blood-sugar issues or diabetes worries. It can also help with constipation since it has laxative and demulcent properties too.

Aloe plants are easy to take care of as a potted houseplant, and difficult to kill once they get to

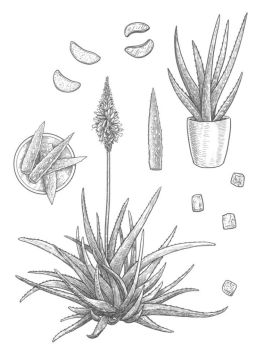

a good size. Tropical desert succulents native to
the Middle East and Africa, they enjoy a lot of sun
but do very well next to a window in most homes,
and require little watering. If you live in a tropical,
coastal or desert climate, you could get away with
growing aloe in your garden – but watch out, it
can be invasive. Any time you have itchy skin, a
superficial burn, dermatitis, dry skin or any other
mild issue with dry or inflamed skin, follow the

lead of other herbalists: harvest a leaf from your aloe plant, cut it open, and place the gel on the affected area.

WARNINGS BEFORE USE: There is little to worry about when using aloe topically. If you experience a reaction, of course, discontinue its use. If you are purchasing an aloe juice or aloe inner leaf gel product (or processing your own gel or juice) for internal use, however, take care that the product is latex free, or that you strain any fibre, latex or leaf matter out of your creation.

The laxative action of the gel or high latex can be very uncomfortable. It can also pose dangers to children and pregnant or nursing mothers, so be careful when buying, processing and using. Read labels for indicators of 'anthraquinone free', 'latex free', 'inner fillet only' or 'free of aloin' (aloin is the name of aloe's trademark anthraquinone compound).

Aloe Sunburn or Windburn Remedy | Tina Sams, Author and Owner of *Essential Herbal* magazine

Says Sams, herbalist and published author of many fantastic herbal healing books on this simple aloe vera recipe: 'I used this on my little one. But at the time, I used lavender essential oil. The hydrosol [or distillate] is much better.'

Hydrosols and distillates are amazing herbal creations that I did not include in this book, as I have very little experience or mastery with them. I would highly recommend getting acquainted with Sams' books and even the back catalogue of *The Essential Herbal* Magazine to learn more about hydrosols. If you plan not to make or use a hydrosol, or do not have lavender essential oil available, using just the aloe is perfectly acceptable.

INGREDIENTS:
¼ cup aloe gel with as few additives as possible
¼ cup lavender hydrosol (or essential oil)

STEP 1 – Place the gel and hydrosol in a measuring cup and blend until it is emulsified and liquid.
STEP 2 – Pour into a 100ml spray bottle and apply liberally. This removes the heat and pain almost on contact.

Adds Sams: 'If you happen to have spent the day snorkelling on a tropical island, chances are there will be giant aloe plants around. Cut a leaf and apply the gel directly to the sunburned areas. With luck, this will save your vacation.'

ANGELICA (Angelica archangelica/Angelica sinensis)

ENERGETICS: Warm and Dry
FLAVOUR: Sweet, Aromatic
PARTS USED: Seeds, Stems, Root (dried only)
BEST PREPARATIONS: Tea or Infusion (seeds or stems); Syrup, Vinegar, Shrub, Tincture, Extract, Bitters
PROPERTIES:
Anti-spasmodic
Carminative
Digestive bitter
Diuretic
Expectorant
Febrifuge
Phytoestrogen
Tussive

Angelica is a tall, spindly, towering flower that has attracted me as a herbalist for many reasons. Admittedly, I have had far fewer encounters with its fragrance and beauty than I would like. It has a wealth of both use and folklore backing it, linked to a shamanic ancestral past of Europe that has been mostly lost through colonization of the continent's distant ancestors (through *Angelica archangelica*). At the same time, in *Angelica sinensis* (also called dong quai), it has long had a hold in eastern Asian healing practices

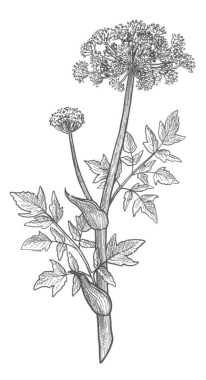

as well, such as in Ayurveda or Traditional Chinese Medicine, and there it has a stronger role as a support herb for women's wellness.

On that note, I have taken up the habit of steering those interested in the Native American and imperilled herb black cohosh for feminine health (owing to its high phytoestrogen content) toward angelica or dong quai instead. Both herbs are also phytoestrogen-rich, have comparable benefits for women's health, and do not suffer the same cultural or environmental issues.

Angelica is a spiritual, digestive and female health remedy. From one herbalist, I learned that the herb was said to be a Celtic favourite for aiding the process of grieving. It also has similar flavourful compounds to herbs I've loved to work with prolifically, such as sweet Cicely, as well as culinary herbs like fennel, anise or lovage, each having at least one thing in common: a sweet liquorice cordial-like flavour. This delightful taste in and of itself is the sign of carminative, anti-spasmodic and digestion-supporting compounds in a herb.

WARNINGS BEFORE USE: If using angelica root (not recommended for beginners), make sure it is thoroughly dried before use, as fresh angelica root – while powerful – can be toxic. Angelica or dong quai's high phytoestrogen levels mean that it interferes with women's hormones. It's probably wise for women to avoid taking it if they are pregnant, trying to get pregnant, or are known to clinically or sub-clinically have excess estrogen. Angelica belongs to the carrot plant family, and quite a few of these plants may also cause photosensitivity or 'photo-dermatitis' – if you eat or touch the plant quite a bit; spending time in the sun may cause rash, welts or advanced sunburn. On that note, angelica is also closely related to some very dangerous wild plants. Stick to buying or cultivating your own and avoid wildcrafting it unless you have the guidance of an expert plant identifier with you.

Angelica Cordial | Ginny Denton, Linden Tree Herbals – Ann Arbor, Michigan

The seeds or stems of angelica on their own make for an excellent aperitif for stimulating the appetite or helping with digestion after meals as a digestif. This exquisite recipe from herbalist Denton takes the classic digestive tonic or bitters to a whole new level.

INGREDIENTS:
Angelica leaves and stems, fresh
Orange slices with peel, fresh
Lemon balm, fresh
Honey (or sugar) to taste
Cinnamon
Cardamom
Allspice
1-pint Mason/Kilner jar with lid
Vodka or brandy

STEP 1 – Fill the jar ⅔ full with fresh chopped angelica leaves and stems.

STEP 2 – Add 3-4 fresh orange slices, peel included.

STEP 3 – Add a handful of fresh lemon balm, chopped medium-fine.

STEP 4 – Fill the jar to the top with good vodka or brandy (up to you) and add 2 dried allspice berries, 2 cardamom pods and a small piece of cinnamon (about 1 inch long).

STEP 5 – Cap the jar, give it a good shake, and infuse for about 4 weeks, shaking the jar every few days. Sweeten with honey to taste.

STEP 6 – Add a tablespoonful to tonic and ice, for a refreshing digestive.

ARNICA (*Arnica montana*)

ENERGETICS: *Warm*
FLAVOUR: *Topical Use Only*
PARTS USED: *Flowers*
BEST PREPARATIONS: *Infused Oil or Basic Salve (see pp. 41 and 47). Or Tea or Infusion (as topical wash only), Poultice, Tincture or Extract (all for topical use on unbroken skin only)*
PROPERTIES:
Analgesic

Discutient
Rubefacient

I've never had the honour of encountering arnica in its natural alpine habitat, even though I've worked with and created preparations from its dried flowers many a time with much success. But if I had, I would have recognized it immediately: a dainty flower with long, pointed, graceful leaves and copious all-yellow daisy-like blooms. It grows in open areas and poor soils at very high

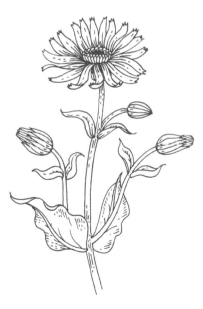

elevations, famously in mountainous areas of
Europe like the Alps and Spanish mountain ranges.
It can only be used topically on unbroken skin (not
on open wounds). When taken internally, it is toxic
and can be lethal.

My experiences with arnica have been many,
and exuberantly positive. Far back in my early
farm days, while helping my partner raise hogs,
I was left with the tough choice of needing to
'manhandle' a large pig who thought I looked and
smelled quite a bit more like food than the food I
was actually giving him. Use of arnica salve, mixed
with a little turmeric, helped immediately melt
away the pain in my bruised hands and knuckles
where the giant pig roughed me up. I can't
recommend arnica enough for topical pain relief
of muscles and bruises. And, working alongside
other pain relievers like CBD or bone-knitters
like comfrey, you have quite the powerful trio and
possibilities with this cheery-looking plant.

WARNINGS BEFORE USE: As emphasized in other
parts of this monograph, absolutely avoid applying
arnica preparations on open skin. That goes for
permeable tissues and mucus membranes, too,
such as sinuses, eyes or mouth. Internal use can
be dangerous, causing heart or breathing issues,
and possibly death. Be very cautious and careful

with use at home; it may be advisable to avoid using arnica at all with young children.

Arnica 'Snake Oil' All-Purpose Salve | Charles 'Doc' Garcia, California School of Traditional Hispanic Herbalism

Garcia, a third-generation *curandero* and herbalist, shares this recipe while mentioning his grandfather's creation of topical remedies from actual snake oil or snake fat (with rattlesnake fat being the most valuable and medicinal). Snake oil had reputed powerful healing properties when used topically on skin. This recipe is also a nod to the 'snake oil' healers of old, who would sell snake oil remedies (such as salves) that were praised as highly effective, but whose reputations became tarnished by bad-intentioned salesmen and irresponsible healers who profited unethically over their own claims, and ruined the reputation of snake oil for quite some time (perhaps forever).

No, you do not have to use actual snake oil or snake fat. Though this specific salve recipe nods to this Native Californian tradition.

INGREDIENTS:
Beeswax
Olive oil
Arnica flowers

Marigold flowers
White sage (aerial parts)
Lavender flowers
Eucalyptus essential oil

See pages 41 and 47 in this book, and follow the infused oil process first – then the salve making process next, all while adhering to the recipe ingredients above. Use the book's recommended ratios of herb to olive oil, and oil to beeswax.

Says Garcia: 'Whether it be snake oil, olive oil... the method is the same...if you use a crockpot (on low) or a slow cooker, it should be ready in four to six hours.' While using a slow cooker or crockpot is not my recommended method in this book, it has worked wonders for Garcia.

When done, 'It is strained with cheesecloth and placed in tins or glass containers. The smell is usually pleasant,' says Garcia.

COMFREY (*Symphytum officinale*)

ENERGETICS: *Cool and Damp*
FLAVOUR: *Topical Use Only*
PARTS USED: *Leaves and Root*
BEST PREPARATIONS: *Poultice (see p. 51). Or Infused Oil, Basic Salve, Strong Cooled Infusion (used as wash or compress), Tincture, Extract*

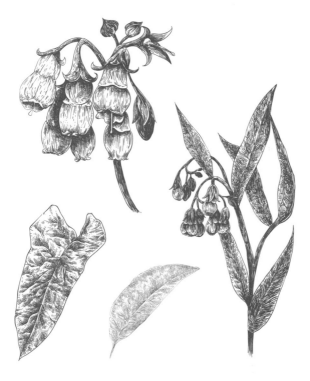

(topical only)
PROPERTIES:
Anti-inflammatory
Discutient
Emollient
Rubefacient
Tissue Regenerator

I remember the first time I 'met' comfrey, watching and helping a herbalist dig up the plant's root to help with an ankle sprain. The flower was...towering. Almost six feet tall, with bright purplish-blue bell-like flowers. When we got to actually digging up the root, the taproot was nearly six feet deep as well. It took quite a bit of effort to extract from the ground, and we still weren't able to pull all of it up. The labour for such a remedy is well worth the effort, though. Few (if any) other herbs rival comfrey's reputation for supporting the body's ability to heal muscle, bone and tendon after an injury when applied to the skin near the injury site. According to research, it can speed up cellular regeneration and healing in a measurable way.

Comfrey is an excellent follow-up remedy to, or a combination remedy with, arnica. Fortunately, it is all right to use on broken skin, though you don't want to consume comfrey internally either (or have it enter the blood stream often, or copiously). The plant is high in pyrrolizidine alkaloids, which in large amounts can be harmful to the liver. The leaves can be poulticed or made into topical salves or oils for healing, though the root is the far superior part to use.

WARNINGS BEFORE USE: There is little to fear from comfrey, even in using the plant as a healer near broken skin (comparative to arnica). However, internal use is not recommended at all due to pyrrolizidine alkaloids and potential liver damage if used excessively or over long periods of time.

Comfrey Root Poultice | Debbie Lukas, Siskiyou Mountain Herbs – Takilma, Oregon

Some herbalists lean toward comfrey topical oils or salves because they make for convenient or sellable products. But most herbalists agree on the science: comfrey root poultice, or even a fresh compress, works best for healing, although leaf salves do have good efficacy.

Says Lukas: 'Comfrey is tricky because of the water content and mucilage.' Indeed, the plant's healing compound that stimulates cellular regeneration (allantoin) is found in the soothing mucilage, which can be partially destroyed when exposed to any heat, even in oil- or salve-making – and the extra water can sometimes make for salves with unpredictable consistency, no matter how much you tweak the ratio of oil to wax.

With a fresh poultice, you sidestep any loss of comfrey's healing compounds. **See p. 51 for further directions on herbal poultice-making.** Or follow Lukas's simple steps right here. As it so happens, Lukas was the very same herbalist who showed me the digging up of comfrey root for my very first comfrey experience, including my first time scrubbing those intimidatingly long (but very healing) roots at her farm in southwestern Oregon.

STEP 1 – Dig up comfrey root. Wash off all dirt with an unimportant dish scrubber or toothbrush. Be sure to pat and air-dry roots before processing.

STEP 2 – Grate the amount of comfrey root you think you will need for the topical area. (Or use other processing methods – see p. 51, poultice section). If you have unused root left over, store it in the fridge or planted in a dirt bucket in a cool location. Avoid grating the entire root and storing, unless you are sure you will use several applications of comfrey poultice within a short period of time (a few days), because the root oxidizes quickly once cut.

STEP 3 – Place the poultice or plaster on the area that needs speedy healing, especially a sprain, bone break or pulled muscle. Cover with a wrap or bandage if desired.

As an extra note, it's best to remove and replace this bandage regularly, at least daily, with a fresh bandage and newly ground poultice applied. In the meantime, place the entirety of your comfrey poultice covered and in the fridge if prepared, or grate more and process, as you need to reapply and replace bandaging regularly until the entire poultice is used up, or until you are satisfied with healing.

GARLIC (Allium sativum)

ENERGETICS: *Warm or Hot*
FLAVOUR: *Spicy, Pungent*
PARTS USED: *Root (bulb and cloves)*
BEST PREPARATIONS: *Consumed Raw or Cooked in Meals; Infused Oil (internal), Vinegar (pickled), Tincture, Extract*
PROPERTIES:
Adaptogen
Alterative
Antibacterial
Antibiotic (raw only)
Anti-diabetic
Antifungal
Anti-inflammatory
Anti-microbial
Anti-parasitic
Antiseptic
Anti-viral
Cardiotonic
Hypotensive

Immunostimulant
Rubefacient
Tonic

If you ever become both a farmer and a herbalist (or just one, or either, really), the day will come – or maybe already has come – where you will be absolutely swimming in garlic. At the same time, you can never have too much garlic around. Garlic is the ultimate culinary herb for both flavour and health benefits. It's not just the pungent, gut-punching flavour that makes it a seminal seasoning the world over. Garlic, both on its own and in dishes, is great for boosting overall health, with a special focus on heart health, immune health and even supporting symptoms of colds, flu and other contagious viruses. The most pungent, hottest varieties are thought to contain the most compounds for stimulating blood flow and immunity, but also boast a near-antibiotic quality when consumed raw (don't worry, there are recipes to help with this). These raw garlic 'doses' may help combat stomach bugs in particular.

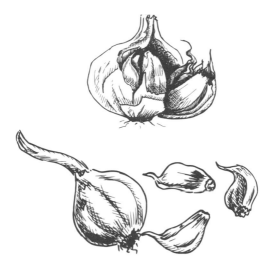

For herbalists or natural health lovers who find themselves consuming quite a bit of store-bought echinacea, consider simplifying things during the winter and sticking to garlic instead. It, too, helps peak immune function in a way that guards against cold and flu symptoms, much like the famous purple coneflower. While it's true that echinacea is most likely commercially grown for the herbal teas or other products you'd buy at natural food stores or supermarkets (and in this case is not overharvested), echinacea is nonetheless an imperilled prairie flower in the wild nowadays, and there's a slight risk that you could be consuming plants from an overharvested population. Plus, it's a Native American medicine that, while effective, is overused and over-associated with immune boosting, while also being overly commercialized and colonized when other less problematic immune boosters are out there.

That's not to say that there's anything wrong with echinacea. Support your local herbalists that prepare these medicines responsibly, through ethical harvesting or even ancestral lineage to the plant's ancient healing use. You can also learn how to harvest the plant ethically yourself. Or, from time to time, give the much more plentiful cultivated alternative garlic a fair swing instead – this is far preferred, especially if you have white colonizer ancestry.

WARNINGS BEFORE USE: No major considerations have been found with garlic, especially if you are only enjoying it for healing occasionally while eating it often. That said, if you are using strong preparations of it for health often, and have cardiovascular issues (and even if you are using it for cardiovascular issues), talk to your doctor or other health professional. Garlic has been known to interact with some clotting medications because its benefits and effects on the heart and blood vessels are so powerful at preventing blood clots, and thus reducing risk of heart attack, stroke and more.

Obviously, exercise caution while processing the raw herb. Its pungency can have a burning, spicy effect that's unpleasant if it gets into the eyes or sometimes even just on the skin. Some people (including myself) have also reported that eating large amounts of raw garlic can cause gastric distress, which can be uncomfortable, but usually goes away on its own.

Garlic Tea for Colds | Maggy Rhein, Fractal Branch Botanicals – Marshall, Arkansas

Maggy Rhein is a small farmer of hemp and creator of healing CBD products in the Ozark Mountains. Alongside her hemp crop rows are many rows of garlic, providing a variety of medicinal remedies for her family and community, some of which are shipped to customers around the country.

Says Rhein of this recipe, 'In 2010, my best friend and I spent two months in Xela, Guatemala, working with a women's weaving cooperative. A tiny vegetarian restaurant was our go-to for a decompression space, and we met the owner, Bonifaz. When one of us came down with a summer cold, he took us to his apartment to prepare this basic but miraculous remedy. I was initially put off by the garlic – 'in my *tea*?!' But a mild variety, and the other ingredients, help set off the savoury flavour and make it an enjoyable experience.'

INGREDIENTS:
1 *knuckle ginger*
1 *cinnamon stick*
1 *large clove garlic*
1 *lemon (for juice)*
Raw honey to taste

STEP 1 – In a small saucepan, heat a cup or so of water, an inch of ginger, chopped, and one whole cinnamon stick.

STEP 2 – Peel one large garlic clove, and dent it with your fingernail several times to bruise and open it (or you could smash it, but this is more personal).

STEP 3 – Once the water has boiled, remove from heat and add garlic and the juice of one lemon. It is important not to boil the garlic so that it preserves some of the healing properties. Cover and let steep for 10 minutes, then pour off into a cup and add raw honey to taste.

HOPS (*Humulus lupulus*)

ENERGETICS: *Cool*
FLAVOUR: *Bitter, Aromatic*

PARTS USED: *Flowers (Cones or 'Strobiles')*
BEST PREPARATIONS: *Tincture, Extract or Bitters
(see p. 62). Or Tea or Infusion*
PROPERTIES:
Anti-spasmodic
Carminative
Digestive Bitter
Emmenagogue
Galactagogue
Nervine
Phytoestrogen
Sedative

A swig from the most bitter IPA beer is a good
introduction to hops – both their flavour and their
effects. With so many different varieties now, the
taste can range from piney to citrusy, zesty, tropical
or just plain bitter. This bitterness explains hops'
virtues as a digestive tonic. It can help jump-start
(or prime) digestion for before or after a meal – but
its other compounds make it a gentle sedative too,
fantastic for helping alleviate stress or anxiety. I
myself love hops tincture and bitters as a flavouring
or adjunct to fruit juices right before bed, to give me
a little extra help before sleep, if sleep seems elusive.
It also has a wonderful flavour when properly
combined with others.

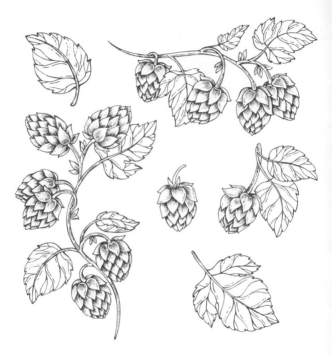

Hop is also noticeably high in phytoestrogens, making it beneficial and therapeutic for women's health or other reproductive or hormonal imbalances in all people. It is a choice I may steer people toward instead of black cohosh, a Native American plant that is imperilled in the wild yet still harvested (and in some cases cultivated) as one of the standard industry supplements for phytoestrogens. Hops have no issues around them, are not imperilled, and are almost exclusively cultivated and plentiful in use as supplements and food all around the world.

WARNINGS BEFORE USE: No major considerations apply to using hops, and they are generally considered safe. Though the phytoestrogen effect is lower and lesser than other herbs, it may be best to avoid using hops while pregnant or breastfeeding, or while trying to conceive – paradoxically, however, they have been used to stimulate breast milk, so the final verdict on this is unclear.

Simple Hops Bitters Recipe

This can go one of two ways. You can make a 'fresh' bitters recipe, or let your cones (preferably completely dried down, but not necessarily) sit in the alcohol menstruum for much longer to technically become a much more potent tincture. While fresh hops can sound alluring – I'm speaking to any beer-brewing readers – I personally prefer drying them completely and processing them into a powder before pouring over the alcohol. This releases the lupulin (hops' active compound and flavour) and tons of flavour right on the spot, not unlike the effect of grinding coffee beans.

I (and many others, I presume) also create any bitters alternative to tinctures in order to take away bitterness and capture a much 'fresher' incarnation of a plant's compounds and flavours (such as with lemon zest). Hop is plenty bitter to start with, however, and is supposed to be. In my observation, by letting it steep longer in a tincture, it doesn't get any more bitter to taste, but it does feel like it gets more potent with time. Meaning: a tincture could still be considered a 'bitters'.

The length of time you decide to let your hops soak or 'macerate' is up to you. Whether you make it into a true tincture or bitters, you're in for a very 'bitter' bitters either way. (See p. 66 for more specifics on bitters creation.)

STEP 1 – Place hops (preferably dried and processed or powdered) in a clean Mason/Kilner jar or other container that is food safe and airtight. Pour the alcohol over the ingredients until they are substantially submerged. (While Everclear or vodka are great choices, if you're strictly going for flavour and not potency, gin is an excellent pairing with hops.)

STEP 2 – Store the jar in a cool, dark place overnight. Give it a good shake a few times, when you remember it. If you like, add other ingredients like grapefruit zest, spruce tips, pine needles or even cedar or juniper berries; all of these pair well with hops.

STEP 3 – The next day, strain the bitters concoction through a fine strainer or cheesecloth into a separate clean container. Store your bitters in a dark place, preferably in dark amber glass containers (blue or green work well too).

Take a few drops or dropperfuls before or after meals to boost digestion or appetite. Or, take a bit before bed, directly on the tongue or in water or juice, to enhance sleep or soothe anxiety.

LEMON BALM (*Melissa officinalis*)

ENERGETICS: *Cool*
FLAVOUR: *Aromatic*
PARTS USED: *Aerial (leaves, tender stems, flowers)*
BEST PREPARATIONS: *Tea or Infusion; Syrup, Tincture, Extract or Bitters*
PROPERTIES:
Analgesic
Anti-spasmodic
Anti-viral
Carminative
Diaphoretic
Digestive Bitter
Nervine

Sedative
Tussive

I have always wondered why lemon balm isn't
a far more famous culinary herb or seasoning,
joining the ranks of relatives or similar plants like
mint, lemon verbena, or lavender, which are such
popular flavours. Lemon balm's taste is divine,
with a very subtle coolness classic to mints (it is
in the mint family) but with a hint of lemony citrus
flavour as well. Even more amazing is lemon balm's
ability to untie the butterflies or knots in one's
stomach – including mine, many a time – with just
a sip from a piping hot tea of the plant, or a few
drops of the tincture or bitters for digestive upset,
stress, anxiety or nervousness. It is also known
to be helpful for soothing the symptoms of mild
depression.

Some herbalists claim that lemon balm has
mild cold-fighting and anti-viral properties, which
makes it an excellent ingredient for topical balm
or salve for cold sores. A hot tea can help bring
on a fever with mild viral illness, say some, as well
as soothe a sore throat. With or without stomach
butterflies, it has awesome digestion-supporting
abilities. Or, if you're suffering the heat on some
scorching summer day, add some sprigs of it to
your favourite iced tea, as a garnish to juice, or

incorporate it with citrus or fruit in a cooling popsicle recipe. Delectable.

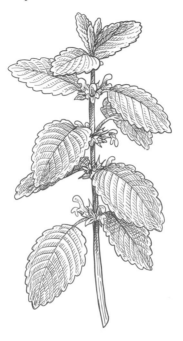

WARNINGS BEFORE USE: There are very few reports of lemon balm being unsafe or having side effects, as it is pretty much categorized with close relatives like peppermint or spearmint, which likewise are safe to use and consume freely. Children and women who are pregnant or breastfeeding can safely consume it. Some herbalists use lemon balm to support hyperthyroidism, which may mean it is best not to use it if you have lower thyroid function.

Lemon Balm Tea | Adrienne Mitchell, Nu Moon Herbals

Mitchell had lots to say about lemon balm – a herb I can tell she's passionate about, and which I truly feel one can't help but be passionate about once you get to know it. She mentioned multiple studies showing that it is effective in healing HSV1 (topical herpes simplex, aka cold sores) and other lesions, and from other herbalists, too, I have heard that it is one of the best and simplest known herbs for the ailment.

Here, Mitchell shares one of her favourite teas featuring lemon balm, saying, 'This blend in a tea can help reduce stress and promote restful sleep.'

INGREDIENTS:
2 tbsp. lemon balm
1 tbsp. chamomile flowers
1 tsp. lavender flowers

Steep this blend in hot water for 5 minutes, then strain. Sit with your tea and inhale the steam, as it contains traces of the essential oils and will aid in relaxation. This is a great time to put intent into your tea, and give it extra direction as to how you want it to aid your body.

Soothing and Centring Everyday Tea | Hillary Schofield, Auriferum – Iowa City

Lemon balm is a popular one. I couldn't resist including an additional recipe for a basic, enjoyable tea from herbalist friend and professional astrologer Schofield. From the spiritual and magickal angle of herbal healing, Schofield as an astrologer had some cosmical tidbits on lemon balm, and this blend as a whole, to share – in the tradition that it was common in ancient times for certain herbal remedies to have astrological significance too.

'The predominant energetics of this blend are of Venus,' says Schofield. 'Venus shows up here as helping to establish equilibrium, smooth out frayed nerves, and bring ease....Looking specifically at lemon balm, in the Western astrological tradition they have most notably been connected with Jupiter and the Sun, reflecting lemon balm's uplifting and vitality-boosting qualities.'

INGREDIENTS:
3 cups spearmint
2 cups lemon balm
Catnip
Chamomile flowers

1 cup red clover
Nettles
Motherwort
Oat straw
Rosebuds and/or petals
Blackberry leaf
Lavender
Skullcap
Marshmallow leaf
½ cup fennel, coarsely ground fresh or powdered
½ cup hawthorn berries
¼ cup orange peel, finely chopped or powdered

Says Schofield, 'All ingredients for this are dried. Amounts shown make about a 3.8-litre batch. You can of course make smaller amounts by dividing the recipe in half (or more). There is a lot of wiggle room with the ratios, and I encourage you to fine-tune it to your tastes. You can also skip some of the herbs if you do not have them, or add others that seem like a good fit. Make it work for you.'

STEP 1 – To brew the tea, I put ¼-½ cup (depending on how much stress relief I am looking for) of the blend in a 1-litre jar and pour boiling water over it. Quickly screw the lid on it and let it sit until it is warm to the touch. One sign I look for is that most of the herbs have fallen to the bottom of the jar, which also makes it easier to pour out – sometimes you may need to burp the lid to allow this to happen.

STEP 2 – I take my mug and place a small strainer over the top and pour the tea in through that. You can also strain it all out into another 1-litre jar and go from there. In the cooler months, I let the herbs continue steeping until I've drunk it all (no longer than 24 hours, typically). In the warmer season, though, it can sometimes go sour by the time I would finish it, so I am more likely to strain it all out at once.

LION'S MANE (Hericium erinaceus)

ENERGETICS: *Damp*
FLAVOUR: *Savoury, 'Umami'*
PARTS USED: *Fruiting Body*
BEST PREPARATIONS: *Tea or Infusion; Syrup; Vinegar; Tincture or Extract*
PROPERTIES:
Adaptogen
Anti-inflammatory (chronic inflammation)
Cardiotonic
Hypotensive
Immunomodulator
Nervine
Neuroprotective

Nootropic
Sedative (mild)
Tonic

Mushrooms were one of many foods I pushed to the edge of my plate as a kid. One day, in my late teens (and during a short fling with veganism), I ate a vegan pizza and was blown away by the flavour. It still managed to be savoury, rich and meaty with absolutely no meat – and it was all because of the mushroom toppings.

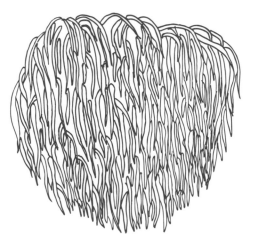

I have found lion's mane and other medicinal culinary mushrooms, such as shiitake or maitake, to hold a unique territory in herbalism and plant-based (or fungi-based) healing because of their 'damp' umami nature. A lot of plants simply cannot do what they do. (To read more about 'damp' herbs and constitutions, energetics and the healing lore behind lion's mane from traditional Asian healing modalities like Traditional Chinese Medicine and Ayurveda, see pp. 178–192.)

At a basic level, lion's mane and other mushrooms contain nutrients we need to be healthy, but which are uncommon in plants – while these same nutrients are present aplenty in animal or meat products. For the vegan, vegetarian, or whole-food plant-based eater, they could be an indispensable food. Meanwhile, when it comes to 'food as medicine', mushrooms like lion's mane are unparalleled immune boosters and inflammation-fighters.

I specifically gravitated toward lion's mane when I was in search of a nervine (nervous system support) healer when I was in my mid-twenties. Having a naturally cold and dry constitution, I sought out a nerve healer – any nerve healer – that would be 'damp' and basically more nourishing to my body than other nervines or adaptogens I was looking at the time. However, most plant nervines are 'dry' and diminishing in nature, even if they were cooling and soothing. How delighted I was to discover lion's mane for my self-care purposes: a mushroom with studies showing it nourishes the nervous system and holistically supports issues surrounding stress, depression, burnout – and may even lower risk of serious neurological issues such as dementia, Parkinson's or Alzheimer's. It also has the added bonus of benefitting the body's fight against inflammation, immune issues, and even supporting heart and blood vessels.

WARNINGS BEFORE USE: Lion's mane is a regularly consumed food around the world and doesn't pose any health hazards. Some people may have mushroom allergies, so if you exhibit these, discontinue its use. In rare instances, lion's mane has been shown to worsen other allergies or asthma. People with liver or other digestive issues may have trouble digesting it.

Lion's Mane Alcohol-Free Extract | Debbie Lukas, Takilma, Oregon

For those with scientific minds, advanced herbalism ambitions, or who want to tap into lion's mane's 'brain power' without the alcohol of tinctures, this recipe (which requires a dehydrator) will be right up your alley.

INGREDIENTS:
500g lion's mane mushrooms (fresh)
170g lion's mane powdered fruiting bodies (dried)
2.4 litres water (preferably filtered)

STEP 1 – Simmer the 500g of lion's mane mushrooms in the 2.4 litres of water for 4 to 8 hours.
STEP 2 – Strain or press out the mushroom material. Return the tea back to a simmer without the mushrooms, and reduce to about 240ml.
STEP 3 – Add the 240ml of liquid to the powdered dry mushrooms, and spread out on a flat cooking sheet or other container that fits inside your dehydrator (and withstands the temperatures – nothing plastic). Dehydrate at 45°C/110°F for about 24 hours, checking regularly.
STEP 4 – Use this dried-down mixture of reduced tea and whole dried lion's mane mushrooms as a daily supplement, add as powder to a hot tea, sprinkle atop foods, or even put into capsules.

MILK THISTLE (*Silybum marianum*)

ENERGETICS: *Cool*
FLAVOUR: *Bitter*
PARTS USED: *Seeds*
BEST PREPARATIONS: *Seeds eaten raw or as seasoning. Or Tea or Infusion, Tincture or Extract*
PROPERTIES:
Alterative
Anti-allergic
Anti-diabetic
Antihistamine
Anti-inflammatory
Carminative
Digestive Bitter
Hepatoprotective

In my personal experience I have only had one encounter with milk thistle: making a preparation and recommending it to a friend who was recovering from substance and alcohol issues for its 'liver-clearing' effect. On the whole, however, I'm more in awe of the plant's enormous wealth of research in favour of its 'detoxifying' and liver-protecting uses, which is fully backed up by experiential and traditional herbalist use. So, I just had to include it, especially as one of the plant world's most powerful liver healers – quite possibly the most powerful liver healer in the plant world.

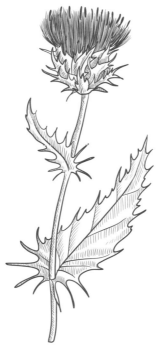

As a herbalist I personally think that just about everyone (not just herbalists) could benefit from a container of milk thistle seeds in their pantry. Because of its amazing effect on the liver (not too unlike agrimony, only more well-studied and possibly more potent) thanks to a compound called silymarin, it can help the body cope with issues of illness to an incredible extent: including excess alcohol consumption, medication overuse, poisoning, animal bites, allergic reactions, a generally unhealthy liver and more. Only a few of these I've been able to witness, while other herbalists have witnessed far more to deem milk thistle a must-have herb for the apothecary. As a bonus, its bitter qualities lend a helping hand to the body when dealing with issues including digestive imbalance, inflammation and allergies.

WARNINGS BEFORE USE: Milk thistle is widely used around the world, sometimes even in conventional medicine situations. It's been shown to be very safe. That said, some would recommend to people with liver issues or disorders to be cautious with the herb and to talk to your doctor about using it beforehand. If you are dealing with any issues related to poisoning, animal bites, severe allergic reactions, overdoses or accidental ingestion of harmful substances or plants, contact an emergency room immediately and do not solely depend on the use of milk thistle.

✿ Harvesting and Drying Milk Thistle Seeds

In late autumn or summer, when all manner of thistle plants go to flower and set their seeds, harvest the tops of your milk thistle plants (whether cultivated or foraged) – ideally with gloves in order to avoid any uncomfortable pricks. Or, alternatively, pick fresh flowers and hang them upside down to dry in a cool, dark place until the tops are dry enough for processing.

Again, preferably wearing gloves (if you're concerned about dried needles – and I would be), carefully coax seeds out of the dried flower pods and set these aside in a dry glass container that can be sealed airtight. Store this container in a dark, dry place. As needed, use milk thistle seed like a medicinal supplement by chewing about one teaspoon of seeds as a dose. This can be done daily to support health, especially liver health. Seeds can also be crushed or ground (possibly even in some pepper grinders) as a seasoning on daily meals for health benefits as well.

MUGWORT (Artemisia vulgaris)

ENERGETICS: *Cool and Dry*
FLAVOUR: *Bitter*
PARTS USED: *Aerial (tender leaves and stems)*
BEST PREPARATIONS: *Tea or Infusion; Infused Oil, Basic Salve, Syrup, Vinegar, Shrub, Tincture, Extract or Bitters*

PROPERTIES:
Anti-microbial
Digestive Bitter
Dream Enhancer
Febrifuge

I have always loved having dreams and exploring what they mean. For the more prolific period

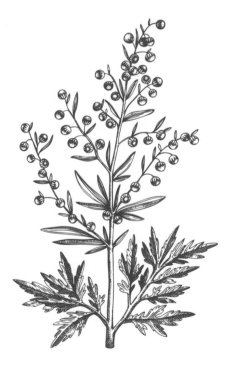

of my life when I worked doing astrological, psychic, and I Ching readings, dream interpretation and 'dream work' were some of my specialties as well: helping people make sense of what their subconscious or unconscious was telling them (or in some beliefs, what the ancestors or spirit world were telling them). Various herbs can aid people in this type of work, with mugwort being one of the most popular; some could call it the poster child 'dream herb' of Western culture.

Many people report also that mugwort can help stimulate not only more vivid dreaming, but lucid dreams as well. A hot tea, which is quite bitter – helped along with some honey sweetening – is one great way to use it. A vinegar may make its bitterness more palatable. Otherwise tinctures, extract or artfully made bitters could lightly stimulate the dreamtime.

Mugwort has other benefits too. A close relative of the highly bitter plant wormwood – of absinthe fame, and also an artemisia family member, like mugwort – the bitterness of mugwort makes its benefits as a digestive healer a fantastic bonus. I would also encourage people to explore mugwort (along with classic Mediterranean garden sage, *Salvia officinalis*) as a replacement herb for 'smudging' as much as possible instead of turning to the Native American herb white sage or estafiate, for multiple reasons; white sage is also a close mugwort relative (*Artemesia ludoviciana*).

Not only is the wild prairie plant white sage overharvested and heavily commercialized, the use of it for spiritual or cleansing purposes can be seen as problematic. (Especially if purchase of the herb goes to a predominantly white-profiting company or entity.) However, mugwort can be burnt just like white sage, and was used for similar purposes among ancient Europeans to cleanse objects and spaces (called 'saining' in Gaelic). This very same smoke from saining, as it purifies, can encourage a more active dream life when you are in the presence of it and inhaling its fragrant fumes…you might just experience interesting dreams later that night.

WARNINGS BEFORE USE: Mugwort is relatively considered safe. Because it stimulates one's dream life and has such a close relation to absinthe psychoactive wormwood, it may be wise to avoid taking it in large doses. Some reported side effects include stimulating uterine contractions, so women may want to avoid internal use during pregnancy, and it is best kept off-limits for children.

🌿 Dried Mugwort Bundle for Smudging

Make your very own mugwort smudge sticks for enhancing dream life, purifying a space, or to add ambience to meditation, mindfulness, ceremony, or a simple serene moment. This can be done by harvesting, drying, and bundling the aerial parts of the mugwort plant.

STEP 1 – Harvest and gather dried mugwort branches. Preference goes to tender-stemmed branches with larger leaves, but if these are scant, use gardening pruners or tough scissors to cut away some of the woodier stems to extract some branches (being careful not to over-harvest from the plant). Ideally, pick branches that are not in flower.

For one full bundle or stick, harvest a bundle of mugwort that fits into the full diameter of the grip of your hand if your fingers were to be completely encircled around the base of the bundle (all four fingers touching the tip of your thumb).

STEP 2 – Tie the bundle together at the base and hang upside down on a line to dry in a cool, dark place until mostly dry but not completely brittle – still pliable for bundling and wrapping.

STEP 3 – Take thin, untreated string (free of plastics or chemicals, as this will be burned while smudging) and methodically loop and wrap the string around the bundle from the very base to the tip, so it makes for a nice and tight bundle that won't fall apart easily. You can do this in parallel wrapping patterns, or crisscross patterns.

STEP 4 – When securely tied and bundled, you're ready to burn your mugwort bundle, starting at the non-stem end. Light with a lighter or matches to emit smoke, smudge, and purify. Make sure to put out any embers completely when not in use.

PINE *(Pinus strobus)*

ENERGETICS: *Cool and Dry*
FLAVOUR: *Aromatic (resinous)*
PARTS USED: *Leaves (needles) – Sap ('resin') or Pollen*
BEST PREPARATIONS: *Tea or Infusion (see p. 34). Or Infused Oil, Basic Salve, Syrup, Vinegar, Shrub, Tincture, Extract, Bitters*
PROPERTIES:
Anti-bacterial
Antifungal
Anti-microbial
Antiseptic
Decongestant
Diuretic

Expectorant
Styptic
Tussive

While going through my two herbalist training programmes in the early 2010s, I was introduced to pine (and especially white pine) as 'the most powerful antimicrobial healer'. Not too long after this I decided to go walking through my home's nearby evergreen woods in search of some white pine sap early one spring, when the evergreen sap would be running. The key is to look for natural gouges or dropped limbs from the pine's tree trunk that would leave an open wound, some time before most leaves and flowers on deciduous plants would be up and blooming. From these wounds, the white pine's sap will flow – a noticeably bright, milky substance, the tree's healing blood itself, designed to clean and close its own wounds. Without harming, cutting or gouging the tree, you can lightly scrape or collect this sticky sap for healing use right off the bark if you can find it. I've used white pine for many things since then, especially for helping with wound healing, keeping wounds clean and protecting against the risk of infection – even as a mouth wash.

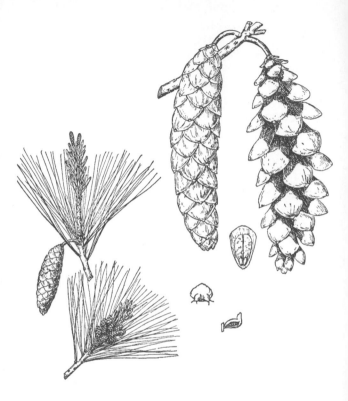

That said, the fresh and tender new pine needles that the tree produces each spring are great for other self-care use too – as are spruce tips, another evergreen tree I've loved to work with and that has similar properties. Either can be used to give things a fabulous gin-like flavour which is supposed to be from juniper, but pine flavour is very similar. When not using the pine resins, fresh tender pine needles from the season's first new growth from the tree can be wonderful to work with too: for creating aromatic cleaners, or even elixirs or bitters that help stimulate the lungs and respiratory tract to deal with coughs, phlegm or congestion.

WARNINGS BEFORE USE: There's little to no reports on side effects from pine that I could find. Since it is mostly a topical remedy for wound cleaning or cleansing, there is very little risk there. Obviously, any sort of skin reaction means you should stop using it, and it could signify an allergy. Pine is high in tannin compounds that are highly astringent; consuming too much internally in flavoured products or other herbal creations (like a tea) could possibly cause some gastric upset, but most people will probably not drink nearly enough to experience that.

White Pine Cordial | Emma Barber, Rhubarb Botanicals in Mt. Vernon, Iowa

While not utilizing white pine's classic wound-healing properties, sometimes the best way to enjoy a herbal remedy is to simply bask in its flavours – just like in this fabulous, tasty cordial recipe. It's a perfect creation to make in the springtime or, really, anytime.

INGREDIENTS:
Fresh white pine needles – approx. 3 cups
2 tbsp. fresh grated ginger or 1 tbsp. dried ginger
Peel & pith of 1 orange
Approx. 600ml of your liquor of choice: gin, vodka, whisky or scotch
250ml honey

STEP 1 – Fill a clean quart-sized glass jar ⅔ full with fresh pine needles.
STEP 2 – Grate 2 tbsp. fresh ginger and add to the jar, or add 1 tbsp. dried ginger.
STEP 3 – Cut the peel of one orange into strips and add to the jar, including the white pith.
STEP 4 – Add other aromatic herbs and spices if you wish. Rosemary, cardamom, cinnamon and/or hawthorn berry would all be excellent choices.
STEP 5 – Pour the honey over the herbs.
STEP 6 – Pour your choice of alcohol over the herbs until the jar is full. Stir well with a clean spoon, then put the lid on the jar and shake well.
STEP 7 – Shake daily or as often as you can remember for one month.
STEP 8 – Strain the liquid from the herbs and decant into a clean jar or fancy bottle.

STEP 9 – Sip your White Pine Cordial neat on chilly winter nights for warming respiratory support, or enjoy it with sparkling water over ice for a refreshing spritzer.

PLANTAIN *(Plantago major/Plantago lanceolata)*

ENERGETICS: *Cool and Damp*
FLAVOUR: *Bitter, Salty*
PARTS USED: *Aerial (tender leaves and stems), Seeds*
BEST PREPARATIONS: *Tea or Infusion; Infused Oil, Basic Salve, (spit) Poultice, Tincture or Extract*
PROPERTIES:
Analgesic
Anti-allergic (topical)
Antihistamine (topical)
Anti-inflammatory
Demulcent
Emollient
Expectorant
Mucilaginous
Styptic

Plantain (no, not the banana relative) has the nickname 'white man's foot' in America for a couple of reasons. Both species listed here came

from Europe on the coattails of white colonizers
and settlers as they arrived in North America,
after which it spread across the land. The other
reason: plantain does appear to flourish the
more you stomp on it. You'll find that the larger,

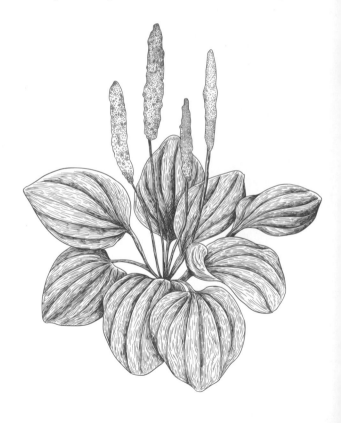

almond-shaped leaf species *Plantago major* prefers disturbed areas or waste sites, especially the more compact the soil is, such as driveways or walkways. *Plantago lanceolata* has somewhat similar preferences, except it does prefer open fields or pastures a little more if you find a nice patch of plantain that looks relatively non-stomped (for safety and sanitary purposes).

If you have a bug bite or bee sting, pick a leaf from the plant and chew it, then place it on the sting (for more specific directions on this 'spit poultice', see below). In most cases the itch or pain will go away immediately. According to herbalists, this effect is optimized by human saliva, though plantain compresses, oils and salves also have benefits.

I myself had the experience of having plantain nearby after an unfortunate encounter with a yellowjacket nest in the Appalachian mountains. Stung at least 10 times, I found that plantain helped quite a bit with the pain for the next few days. Besides bee stings and itching, however, plantain has an emollient and demulcent action somewhat similar to aloe or comfrey, and can be eaten or taken internally as well as topically. You can also use it in a topical salve to help remove poison ivy oils right after contact, to soothe a sunburn, or to temporarily stop the bleeding of a wound.

As food, I've used raw leaves in smoothies with a focus on cooling detoxification support internally, but I could see a plantain tea helping with raw, unproductive and dry coughs. Of note, plantain is a close relative of *Plantago ovata*, or psyllium seed. The leaves do have a mild laxative effect, and most likely, the seeds even more so. (Though use with caution and at your discretion – I cannot guarantee this is a safe or comfortable experience.)

WARNINGS BEFORE USE: Plantain leaf is probably one of the safest and most harmless remedies I've come across. Regardless, be cautious: test it on your skin to see if you have any dermatitis reaction or allergy before chewing it or using it topically. Internally, eating large amounts of plantain could have a laxative effect...this may just be more undesired than unpleasant.

❦ The Infamous Plantain Spit Poultice

Almost every novice herbalist (including myself, when I was just learning) learns the plantain spit poultice, as it is one of the easiest, quickest and most effective tricks to learn for bug bites and bee stings. The relief is immediate, the steps are simple...and the original 'recipe' is attributed to no one. It's just an old-timey herbalist trick.

STEP 1 – Pick a plantain leaf, and rinse it with cool water first if you like.

STEP 2 – Chew the leaf; this is essential, as salivary enzymes are key to 'awakening' the antihistamine effects.

STEP 3 – Spit or place the chewed poultice on the bug bite or sting. You should feel relief from pain or itching in seconds. Rinse away the plant matter once symptoms are gone.

STINGING NETTLE *(Urtica dioica/Laportea canadensis)*

ENERGETICS: *Drying, Slightly Warming*
FLAVOUR: *Bitter, Salty*
PARTS USED: *Aerial (tender leaves and stems), Seeds*
BEST PREPARATIONS: *Tea or Infusion; Syrup, Vinegar, Tincture or Extract*
PROPERTIES:
Adaptogen
Anti-allergic
Antihistamine
Anti-inflammatory
Decongestant
Diuretic
Tonic

Anyone who is new to the woods (especially those who didn't grow up near woodlands) has been fearful of stinging nettle and its itching, burning pain upon contact. That includes me, a suburban-raised kid who, though I loved to play in nature, grew up in the southwestern United States and didn't encounter it much until I was an adult. I heard horror stories about stands of it in deeper woods up in the mountains, but never encountered them. Once I became a Midwesterner (where nettle can absolutely fill a forest understory) and travelled around the country more, my encounter came. How ironic that a herb that causes burning pain and dermatitis can be a fantastic plant-based inflammation-fighting food. Apparently, the histamine in its needles may be responsible for this.

Eating it regularly may not only help support inflammation from things like arthritis pain, but also sinus inflammation and congestion. Stinging nettle is also incredibly high in vitamins and minerals for combating fatigue, and that goes for wood nettle (*Laportea canadensis*), the native species to the United States, as well. I myself have experienced a sort of stimulating and clearing energy afterward when consuming it regularly, which I can only credit to its amazing nutrients. This is why stinging nettle has long been recommended for or administered to

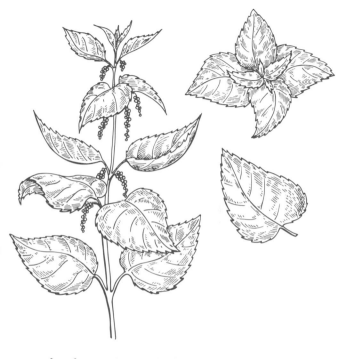

people who are in need of more energy and less inflammation in their lives – especially those dealing with spring or seasonal allergies. After some time eating and enjoying stinging nettle as a food or medicine, when I've happened to get 'nicked' by some out in the wild, somehow its sting doesn't smart as much for me...and maybe that's due to my appreciation of it.

WARNINGS BEFORE USE: Mind the sting while harvesting. Sensitivity to it varies among different people, so use sleeves and gloves while harvesting if you don't want to get stung. Nettle is considered very 'drying' because it is a diuretic, so avoid overusing or overeating it – this can be a little hard on the kidneys and have an opposite nutritive effect in loss of minerals through more frequent urination. There are some concerns that nettles can stimulate uterine contractions, so pregnant women may be wise to avoid it.

Black Strap Nettle Syrup

This is my go-to preparation and method for taking nettles daily for their energetic and nutritive benefits, rather than drinking the bitter infusion daily. The addition of molasses, also high in vitamins and minerals, makes it an even more powerful and pleasant tasting tonic 'supplement'. For more guidance on syrup making for this, see pp. 54–57.

INGREDIENTS:
Dried (or fresh) stinging nettles (at least 1 cup)
550-850ml honey (preferably organic; raw is OK)
420-570ml black strap molasses
Water

STEP 1 – Fill a small to medium pot with water. Bring to a gentle simmer, then add the nettles to create the initial infusion. Cover. Let it simmer for a while, until the water is a very dark green. You can leave it to simmer, or just leave it on low heat. The sludgier-looking, the better (more vitamins/minerals). You may add more water if too much evaporates, and infuse as long as you like. It may take a while.

STEP 2 – Strain out the herb from the infusion and put the liquid in a new, clean pot. Add the honey and bring it up to a simmer again.

STEP 3 – At this point, you are 'simmering down' your syrup to the consistency you like. This may also take a while. Stir it a bit from time to time. Some syrups can be runnier, with more water content, others can be a bit thicker; it just depends upon the length of simmering. A couple of notes: syrups are runnier at a higher temperature, so it will be a bit thicker when it has cooled. Also, the black strap molasses may increase thickness.

STEP 4 – Once the syrup has reached the desired consistency, add the molasses to the mixture and stir while it is still hot. Let cool.

STEP 5 – Add the cooled Black Nettle Syrup to a container, preferably glass and amber-tinted. Make sure to store syrup in fridge when not in use.

SUMAC (*Rhus typhina*, other *Rhus* species)

ENERGETICS: *Cool and Dry*
FLAVOUR: *Sour, Bitter*
PARTS USED: *Berries*
BEST PREPARATIONS: *Tea or Infusion (cold infusion best for flavour); Syrup, Vinegar, Shrub, Tincture, Extract or Bitters*
PROPERTIES:
Anti-diarrhoeal
Anti-microbial
Antiseptic
Astringent
Diaphoretic
Digestive Bitter
Diuretic
Tonic

As a kid in the Southwest, I would play in a small stand of sumac bushes thinking they were a jungle or tropical forest, mostly because of their exotic appearance. As an adult studying herbalism much later in the Midwest, I would look upon those graceful shrubs, with their blazing sunset foliage in autumn and bright red berries, and wonder: does this favourite childhood plant of mine, native to North America, have any healing benefits? I was delighted when I found out the answer was yes, not only as a vitamin C-rich infection fighter and microbe killer for oral issues, but also for treating common colds and flu.

If you've explored eastern Mediterranean cooking, you've no doubt heard of powdered sumac berry in za'atar, a Lebanese cooking spice. It can be described as earthy, sour, a little bit fruity and very cooling. As for the native species from North America, sumac berries (especially

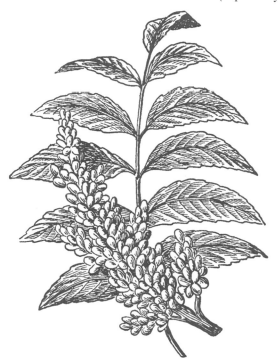

staghorn sumac, the most flavourful variety native to the United States) are used to make delicious sumac-ade, a beverage of Native American origin. I quickly fell in love with sumac because of its beauty, the childhood connections, and its wonderful, sour flavour – and also because of how good it is for health and healing. It is strongly astringent and anti-microbial (especially the less flavourful but more bitter species of smooth sumac, *Rhus glabra*); and with the plant's help, I was able to speed up my healing after wisdom-tooth surgery, and fight off strep throat.

Even more amazingly, I recommended the plant to a friend, who reported that it helped him sidestep root canal surgery. (Of course, be sure to consult with a dentist about tooth surgery, and don't rely on plants – my friend was a lucky example.) Rich in tannins in the berry drupes' stems and bark, sumac may also support digestive regularity and help fight stomach bugs or pathogens, thanks to its anti-diarrhoeal and anti-microbial properties.

WARNINGS BEFORE USE: Few concerns surround sumac, and it can be consumed safely by just about anyone in fairly plentiful culinary or healing amounts. It is a tannin-rich plant, so eating or drinking excessive amounts of the berry may cause some gastric upset. If harvesting in the wild, know the difference between culinary or medicinal sumacs and poison sumac. The poisonous relative has bright white berries and grows in swamplands; make sure you know how to tell them apart, as poison sumac can cause painful rashes.

Sumac-Ade | Nico Albert, Burning Cedar Indigenous Foods

Nico Albert of the Cherokee Nation shares this recipe, which allows users access to the easiest, most flavourful and arguably one of the most medicinal (and enjoyable) sumac preparations out there – for which we have indigenous knowledge to thank. Albert's work with Burning Cedar Indigenous Foods aims to restore these same healing and foodways that have been lost through colonization and co-opting: the very foundation to healing I speak of in this book's introductory sections, specifically in 'How Do Herbs Work?'.

Sumac-ade is not strictly a tasty beverage, but I dare say it's the most superior method for extracting sumac's healing qualities and flavours (though I've enjoyed it as a bitters). Technically, it could be termed a 'cold infusion'. See pp. 36–38 for more guidance on creating herbal infusions.

INGREDIENTS:
4-5 drupes (clusters of sumac berries)
Cold water
Sweetener of choice (agave nectar, honey, stevia)

STEP 1 – Rinse drupes under cold water to remove any dirt, debris or insects. Rest assured, however, that the berries are just fine to use for infusion if you're concerned about any microbial activity (sumac is strongly anti-microbial).

STEP 2 – Place rinsed berries into a clean dish or pot filled with room-temperature water. One sumac drupe will strongly infuse around 1 cup of water, so keep that in mind as you add your water (to guarantee stronger flavour, however, feel free to add more).

STEP 3 – Agitating the berries and drupes will speed up the extraction and add flavour. Simply use a potato masher, large spoon or even meat tenderizer to crush the berries a bit before letting the passive extraction happen.

STEP 4 – Let the berry extraction steep for at least a few hours or even overnight. The longer, the better.

STEP 5 – Once satisfied with appearance and flavour, strain out the berries and twigs from your sumac-ade. You can use a fine strainer, cheesecloth or whatever you prefer – the finer the better. My

favourite method is to use a French press.
STEP 6 – Pour the strained sumac into a glass and sweeten to taste. I like to drink it cold, or over ice, to hail the transition from late summer into autumn.

VALERIAN (Valeriana officinalis)

ENERGETICS: Cool
FLAVOUR: Bitter, Aromatic, Slightly Sweet
PARTS USED: Root
BEST PREPARATIONS: Decoction, Poultice, Syrup, Vinegar, Shrub, Tincture, Extract or Bitters
PROPERTIES:
Antiseptic
Digestive Bitter
Nervine
Sedative
Styptic

I love valerian – and not just because the plant has helped lull me to sleep many a time. The herb has a strong connection to Celtic roots and Druidic practice that has been lost over time, and it once was esteemed (and still is among a few, I'm sure) as a ceremonial and magickal herb – and, surprisingly to some, as a wound cleaner and healer, too. It is a sedative, so much so that it could easily be called a narcotic – but it is hardly intense enough to become addictive or habit-forming, which is why it can be easily found and sourced in tea form.

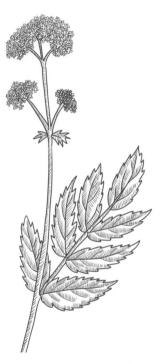

Compared to other sedative herbs like hops and lemon balm, its effects are far more palpable immediately after taking it. Whereas one minute I thought I couldn't sleep, a few moments later I would find my eyelids to be heavier. My very first time taking valerian root was in a concoction of other herbs, and its effects surprised me. I didn't believe that something botanical and natural could knock me out so quickly. I woke up, a little embarrassed, in a room that was now empty of the people that were in it before, realizing I had fallen asleep in a soft chair in the middle of a gathering. A strong testament to its effectiveness – and it hasn't failed me since. People should not underestimate its other ancient uses, for digestion and as a wound healer, though these are less potent compared to other plants, like angelica or pine. That said, it far outweighs these other categories as a sleep-supporting herb.

WARNINGS BEFORE USE: When used conservatively, occasionally and as directed, valerian is a perfectly safe and effective herb for sleep. However, among some people it has been reported that valerian can have the opposite effect: giddiness, alertness and hyperactivity. Of course, if this happens to you, seek out a different sedative herb to help you, such as lemon balm or hops.

Avoid consuming high amounts of valerian root tea, extracts or even supplements, no matter how much you struggle with getting to sleep. This can cause nausea, vomiting, confusion, headaches, dizziness, giddiness and all sorts of unpleasant side effects. It's generally recommended to avoid using valerian in children, or in women who are pregnant or nursing.

Basic Valerian Bitters Recipe

Valerian is a tricky herb, as its flavour is unpleasant to some, whether in tea or tincture form. But this doesn't make its sleep-enhancing effects any less desirable. I recommend adding a little sweet and acidity to a bitters recipe featuring valerian (see p. 66 for more info on bitters creation) or, inversely, to flavour an already fully potent tincture.

INGREDIENTS:
Valerian root (preferably fresh, though slightly dried is OK)
Citrus zest of choice (orange, grapefruit, lemon or lime)
Sweetener of choice (honey, agave or syrup)

STEP 1 – Place valerian root, fully processed (chopped or ground), in a clean Mason/Kilner jar or other container that is food safe and airtight. Pour alcohol over the ingredients until they're substantially submerged.

STEP 3 – Store the jar in a cool, dark place – only overnight if you would like subtly flavoured, low-potency valerian bitters. Or, if you want very bitter, high-potency valerian tincture, let it steep or macerate for at least a month. Give it a good shake a few times whenever you remember it.

STEP 4 – After an overnight steep (or when

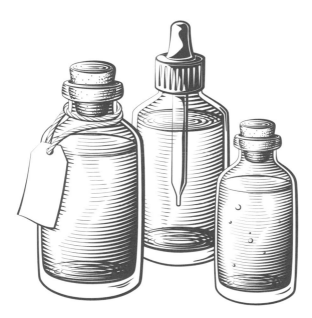

a month is up), strain the bitters concoction through a fine strainer or cheesecloth into a separate clean container.

STEP 5 – Add up to 1 tablespoon of your zest of choice to the strained tincture of bitters, as well as a sweetener to taste. Let this newly flavoured valerian concoction sit overnight, or around 12 hours.

STEP 6 – Remove or strain out the zest. Taste test for sweetness and acidity, then add zest or sweetener until the desired balance of flavours is achieved. When done, store in a dark place, preferably in dark amber glass containers (blue or green work well too).

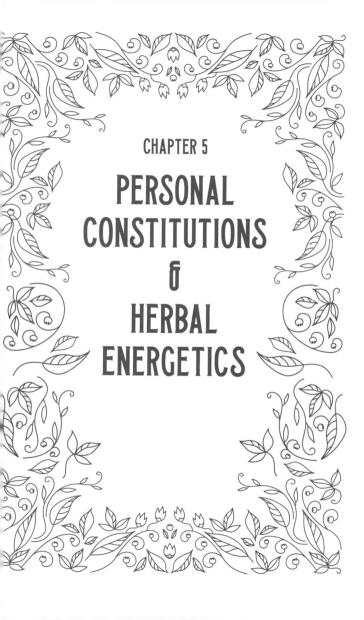

CHAPTER 5

PERSONAL CONSTITUTIONS & HERBAL ENERGETICS

When first studying herbalism and the specifics of each herb, the idea of having to memorize *every* single detail about the plant and what it may do can be overwhelming (and when you go about it that way, it can be a real task). Herbal properties can seem random at first – that is, until you get introduced to herbal energetics and energetic constitutions.

Herbal energetics can help key you into the overall effects of a herb at a quick glance, and even categorize different herbs together, helping you remember their specific effects simply by association. It certainly helped me (and still does), as well as many other home herbalists and practitioners. Energetics aren't always included as sections to intro herbalism books for healing, but I couldn't resist it since it has been a boundlessly helpful tool.

As you read the monographs of different herbs in the previous section – and through the next section on Tastes of Herbs – you will notice the modifiers 'warm', 'hot', 'cold', 'cool', 'dry', 'damp' and 'moist'. These are a nod to the classic systems of herbal energetics that we have to thank for this type of understanding, specifically Ayurvedic medicine and Traditional Chinese Medicine, which generally have more complex systems of herbal or alternative health energetics (the section in this book being only a simplified version). That's not to say there aren't other basic energetic approaches to using herbs for healing found in other cultures, including in modern Western Herbalism.

You'll also notice that energetic qualities don't just apply to the herbs...they apply to people too. Do you think you are a warm, dry person? Or maybe cool and damp? (Yes, you can be more than one – though you can't be dry and damp or hot and cold at the same time, of course.) **Taking cool herbs if you have a warm constitution, or dry herbs if you have a damp constitution, for example, is said to bring your body and health back into balance and holistic homeostasis.** Following this categorical way of thinking and determining the best remedies for yourself can be extremely helpful, especially if you don't know where to start finding the remedies that could help you, or you're uncertain of your 'allies'.

Categorizing herbs can also be 'elemental', correlating to earth (cool/cold), fire (hot/warm), wind (dry) and water (damp). That said, using warm/cool/damp/dry with energetics better taps into the wisdom and knowledge of most herbal energetic approaches. You may already be intuitively drawing upon the basic idea: if herbs are cool or cold, they could be beneficial to warm people or warm conditions, and vice versa. And you'd be right. The same goes for dry remedies for damp constitutions or conditions, and this forms the basis of 'energetics'. Keep in mind: this is only a guiding principle for using herbs – it's not a hard and fast rule or something to live by. Herbs (and people) simply cannot be 'over-categorized'. In many instances, you may find yourself drawn to using a herb that simply doesn't follow energetic 'rules', or that your own elemental constitution doesn't seem to apply to (such as simply looking for sleep- or dream-enhancing herbs, like valerian and mugwort). But, when you have no idea where to start, energetics can help.

Are herbal energetic categories rigid and static? Absolutely not. In fact, as you do more research on herbalism, you'll find that herbalists and different modalities can have varying opinions on the energetics of certain herbs – whereas the energetics of other herbs are not up for debate (aloe being damp and garlic being hot, for example). While herbal energetics are something that clinical or professional herbalists are more apt to use, I've included a basic breakdown because I firmly believe that they are helpful to anyone getting acquainted with herbs for healing

– even if it's just at home while making your own preparations and formulas, or getting to know your health and self-care needs. It can also just be a fun way to explore herbalism in general.

Disclaimer: This section is not designed to help you diagnose issues in yourself or others, nor to prescribe natural remedies for yourself or others – especially for serious symptoms or health conditions. It is simply meant to be an educational guide to understanding herbs and the possibility of using them in self-care.

꩜ The warm/hot constitution | qualities | health conditions

Identifying a warm or hot person is probably the easiest and most recognizable process in energetics. It's also the easiest to recognize in most of the classic warming herbs. Someone who seems 'fiery' is most likely to be a 'hot' person, but they can also be defined by tending towards inflammatory issues, a lot of energy, a higher metabolism and higher blood pressure. Everything about the hot constitutions is a bit 'over-stimulated'. But keep in mind: energetics only represent a spectrum. Someone can lean closer to having hot constitutional issues, but have cold issues too.

Hot-natured or warming herbal remedies are not what someone with a warm constitution would be after, however; remedies of a cooling nature (listed below) are what they may need. Many of these remedies have slight to moderate sedative properties, to let cooler heads prevail. They slow down metabolism, reduce over-stimulated circulation, energy, mood and more. If inflammation is an issue especially, cold remedies are just the thing, no matter what their constitutional complexion.

Remember: this description of warming/hot energetics does not limit what hot-natured herbs are fully capable of; it is just a guide.

TRAITS OF A WARM/HOT CONSTITUTION

Higher cold tolerance
Gets warm or hot easily
Prone to fevers
Common issues with inflammation (rosacea, reddened skin etc.)
Digestive issues (esp. diarrhoea, high acidity, overactive digestion)
High blood pressure
Strong complexion
Higher metabolism
Inflammatory pain
High energy
Quick to anger or annoy, hot-tempered

▶ *Warm or Hot Health Conditions:*

Burns (sunburn, first- and second-degree
burns etc.)

Muscle fatigue from overuse

Diabetes

Inflammatory conditions

Inflammation, swelling and associated pain

Some autoimmune conditions

Fevers

Hyperacidity

Allergies (with inflammation symptoms)

Ulcers

Heartburn

Hyperthyroidism

▶ *Classically Cold or Cool Herbs and
Remedies (best for hot conditions and
constitutions):*

Agrimony (see p. 99)

Aloe vera (see p. 104)

Comfrey (see p. 118)

Cucumber

Gentian

Hibiscus

Hops (see p. 128)
Nopal cactus
Lemon balm (see p. 133)
Mint (topical)
Pine (see p. 152)
Plantain (see p. 157)
Sumac (see p. 166)
Valerian (see p. 171)

❦ The cold/cool constitution | qualities | health conditions

Compared to those with heated constitutions, cold or 'cool' people may be hard to spot. Their issues can be related to a *lack* of immune response or circulation, which often manifest as low energy, sensitivity to cold and issues with pain and sluggish bodily processes. Emotionally, the cool constitution is generally more level-headed – maybe too level-headed, to the point of avoiding emotion, where it manifests as physical pain and issues instead. Instead of inflammatory pain, like in the warm constitution, cold people may struggle with things like cramping, fatigue and numbness in tissues.

The warming remedies below may be perfect for these people, helping jump-start a slow immune system or circulation issues. They help

accomplish what comes naturally to people
with a hot complexion: they warm the body,
stimulate blood flow, bring on a fever or heat,
improve circulation, increase metabolism, ramp
up digestion and bring a strong spike in immune
response, especially if an inflammatory immune
response is needed. This is perfect for colder or
cooler people.

TRAITS OF A COLD/COOL CONSTITUTION

Lower cold tolerance
Gets cold easily
Slow or sluggish digestion
Poor circulation and numbness issues
Low blood pressure
Pale complexion
Digestive issues (esp. constipation, slow
digestion, cramping, etc.)
Lower metabolism
Cramping pain
Low energy

▶ *Cold or Cool Health Conditions*:

Muscle fatigue and pain from lack of use
Cramping (from lack of circulation)
Arthritis
Joint pain

Infection or sepsis (STAPH, MERCA etc.)
Cold extremities
Hypothyroidism

▶ *Classically Warm or Hot Herbs and Remedies (best for cold conditions and constitutions):*

Angelica (see p. 110)
Arnica (see p. 114)
Cinnamon
Cloves
Citrus (zest)
Elecampane
Garlic (see p. 123)
Ginger
Ginseng
Horseradish

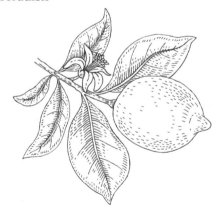

Hot peppers (cayenne, habanero etc.)
Mustard (seed)

❦ The dry constitution | qualities | health conditions

People with dry (also called airy or 'windy')
constitutions are characterized by tension,
dryness, anxiety and an overall lack of health and
vitality. Tissues are tight and tense, and their
minds tend to be too. Dryness due to allergies or
respiratory issues is possible – and of course, dry
skin is too. Being 'dry' has a strong correlation to
the nervous system being depleted, but it can be a
general wasting away of the body with weight loss,
hair loss, dehydration, kidney issues and a parched
appearance or complexion. You can be a warm and
dry person or a cold and dry person, as the dry
constitution overlaps with these temperaments.
Or you may simply have a dry condition that needs
damp remedies.

Dry people need damp remedies plus
some warming or cooling, depending on other
dimensions to their constitution. Such remedies
bring much-needed moisture and nutrients to
those who struggle with dryness – but they would
slip right through the holes for someone with a
damp constitution. (For someone who is already

damp, dampening would be their bane.) Damp herbal remedies nourish the nervous system to soothe anxiety, relieve tension, moisten skin and tissues, and bring a deficient body back into balance. They also tonify the kidneys, which can be central to the dysfunction in dryness in some cases. If you have a windy or airy disposition, your body will welcome an abundance of nutrients and moisture, ideally soaking it right up.

TRAITS OF A DRY CONSTITUTION

Dry skin, eyes, tissues
Easily dehydrated
Difficulty sweating
Very tense (muscular and nervous)
Prone to anxiety
Doesn't cope well with stress
Spacy, cognitive issues
Extreme tension but can't relax (fatigue)
Weakness
Thin physique or weight loss
Hair loss
Tends to skip meals, low appetite

▶ *Dry Health Conditions:*
Anxiety disorders
Migraines

TMJ and bruxism
Some autoimmune conditions (esp. nervous)
Asthma
Dry respiratory conditions (e.g. COPD)
Dry skin/dermatological problems
Indigestion
Kidney issues
Dry cough
Muscle spasms and cramps
Hormone deficiency
Nutrient deficiencies

▶ *Classically Damp Herbs and Remedies*
   (best for dry conditions and constitutions):

Aloe vera (see p.104)
Burdock
Cleavers
Comfrey (see p. 118)
Hollyhock
Lion's mane (see p. 139)
Marshmallow
Plantain (see p. 157)
Shiitake

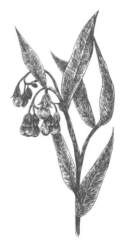

✺ The damp constitution | qualities | health conditions

It can be hard to put your finger on or define the true nature of a 'damp' person. While they can be characterized by an 'excess' of something, that's not always easy to pinpoint – though excess weight or obesity can be a factor (but not always). A sense of stagnancy and an 'overloaded' constitution, in need of cleansing or detoxifying, is more accurate, and may be traced to the liver or gut health. Looking at flesh, skin tone or complexion may be a better way to identify dampness: if there seems to be sagginess, a lack of tone or pallor, and a lot of water retention, there is probably some excess to be found. Think of damp constitutions as waterlogged, or sluggish.

In that case, you can bet that you're dealing with someone who is overly damp and, as such, they'll be in need of drying or tonifying remedies to get things moving and 'aired out' again. The liver is a great organ to target, as are the gut and intestines, which will be in dire need of astringency and tonifying in order to recover their balance.

Remedies of a drying nature can be incredibly powerful and restorative for damp people and conditions. They help tonify skin and cleanse tissues, detox the liver and get fluids in the

body moving and expelled to remove waste and
stagnation that has been hanging around too long.
Many of them are great at kick-starting the liver to
get it into gear to help damp issues too.

TRAITS OF A DAMP CONSTITUTION:

Weepy skin, eyes, tissues
Sweats easily
Prone to weight gain
Prone to inactivity/lack of exercise
More phlegm and mucus
Sad or stagnant emotionally (depression
possible)
Saggy or doughy complexion
Clammy skin
Low energy, lethargic
May have higher appetite

▶ *Damp Health Conditions:*
Depression
Damp respiratory conditions
Liver issues
Edema (water retention)
Overactive bladder
Wet cough
Lymphatic congestion
Low immunity

Chronic diarrhoea
Hormone excess
Leaky gut and Crohn's disease

▶ *Classically Dry Herbs and Remedies (best for damp conditions and constitutions):*

Cranberry
Dandelion
Stinging Nettle (see p. 160)
Parsley
Sumac (see p. 166)
Usnea

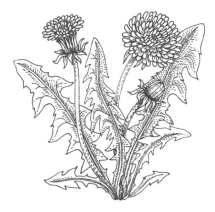

CHAPTER 6

THE TASTES OF HERBS

This next section is one of my favourite realms to explore with herbalism, and has informed me on a lot of my craft. Newcomers may be put off by the idea that some herbs just don't taste good – and that can be true – but whatever the flavour, it shouldn't be a mystery to new herbalists that, in many cases, flavour has a lot to do with a patron herb's healing properties (and on that note, some herbs really do taste wonderful).

Below is a guide to the different tastes you can experience while caring for the self with herbs. **Herbs are not just bitter.** If you've been fortunate enough to explore a few already, then you've no doubt also encountered herbs that are aromatic, salty or even sour – but they don't stop there. Many of these flavours have significance, and can correlate to the different 'energetics' of herbs, which you can explore in the energetics chapter.

Each flavour section will contain an extensive list of healing herbs that fall under that flavour category; there may be more than one opinion about the true flavour nature of a herb, or it may fall under more than one category. For deeper insights into the healing benefits of certain herbs, be sure to explore the monographs. (Note that strictly topical herbs, like arnica or comfrey, obviously do not have a flavour profile associated with their healing benefits, and you won't find them here.)

BITTER

Most herbs you taste will be bitter – and that's not a bad thing. The majority of herbs have bitter properties even if they have another characteristic flavour profile that is more noticeable. Though it may be many people's least favourite flavour, bitterness is arguably the most healing of all the taste sensations, and for many reasons. For one, research shows that the bitter flavour (typically caused by naturally occurring alkaloids) has an immediate effect on the body, causing a chain reaction of physiological responses that are beneficial to you – though in excessive amounts, they can be less good for you. In fact, the body's response to the bitter flavour is theorized to be a response to possible poisons (since most plant poisons are bitter alkaloids).

Thankfully, most bitter foods and herbs (when used correctly) are far from poisonous – quite the opposite! Bitter alkaloid constituents in plants kick-start the digestive system to work harder, which amps up digestive function. Here you have the underlying mechanism behind the before (or after) dinner mint, aperitif or digestif:

just the right amount of bitter helps keep things moving and digesting. It also helps regulate blood sugars, keeping them from peaking or dropping precipitously. This is an amazing ally for diabetics and pre-diabetics, or to curb the effects of too many sweets.

Gently tricking the body into thinking it's been poisoned can be an impressive catalyst for healing. And it's not as terrible as it sounds. This effect happens every time you eat healthy leafy greens, roasted asparagus, orange zest or even drink a cup of coffee. Some bitter compounds are called terpenes, and these can have stimulating (or soothing) effects on the nervous system, as in the case of mugwort, valerian and hops – and all are mildly sedative. In terms of energetics (refer to the energetics section), the bitter flavour generally has a drying effect.

Aloe vera (see p. 104)
Artichoke
Burdock
Citrus (peel)
Cucumber
Dandelion
Elecampane
Gentian
Hops (see p. 128)

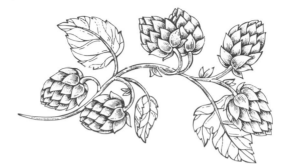

Milk thistle (see p. 144)
Mugwort (see p. 147)
Valerian (see p. 171)

SWEET

Can sweetness be healing? If you're eating lots of sugar, no. Still, certain herbs have a distinctly sweet flavour upon first taste, and they have unique qualities too. When we bite into something sweet, the appetite is stimulated immediately. Digestion slows, and blood sugar spikes (for a small rush of energy – though this is much less the case with non-sugar sweetness). Generally speaking, more food is eaten while metabolism slows down. This can have its benefits – namely, if your body is hungry for a sudden energy burst to keep it going. Sweetness detected in most herbal remedies, however, is thanks to phytochemicals called polysaccharides that help respiratory function, immunity and more. These may not be as distinct as sugary sweetness, but they are sweet nonetheless, and hit the same receptors. What's most notable about the sweet flavour is its ability to 'moisten' and encourage the body to produce more mucus. People with dry constitutions, and with especially dry airways or respiratory issues, benefit from these classic sweet herbs, and many of them have marginal benefits too (such as boosting immunity and digestive function).

Angelica (see p. 110)
Anise
Echinacea
Fennel
Ginseng
Liquorice root

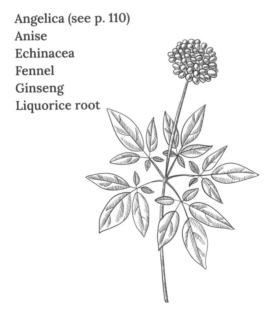

New England aster
Red clover (flower)
Sweet cicely (anise root)
Sweetfern
Violet (flower)

SALTY

The purpose of some herbal tastes isn't to boost digestive, respiratory or any other specific function. Sure, they may be able to address some of these things. But in the long run, they help everything holistically. That said, some herbs have an easy job, acting pretty much like a vitamin supplement or tonic. In short, they're purely nutritive.

When it comes to flavour, one of the quickest ways to recognize the nutritive quality of a herb is through the function of salty taste. It's a sure sign that there are minerals present, including iron, magnesium, sodium, zinc and more – important nutrients. The salt taste function accomplishes the opposite of bitter: it signals that this is a rich, tasty, nutritive food that will be good for you when there isn't too much of it (when too salty, the taste buds will be overwhelmed and reject it). The right amount of salty increases appetite and encourages you to eat more while helping the body modulate electrolyte levels and hydration, which are important for healthy lymphatic and immune function.

We all know that salting food helps enhance the flavours of meals too. That's because of the salt function's appetite-encouraging effects. Most of the herbs below have a preponderance of saltiness, but include some bitterness as well. The result: rich nutrition that is quickly assimilated by a bitters-optimized digestive system. Most herbalists agree that salty herbs tend to have a cooling effect. They can be either moistening or drying too, depending on the herb.

Brassica/Cruciferous vegetables
Chickweed
Cleavers
Hollyhock
Horsetail
Marshmallow
Nasturtium
Oats

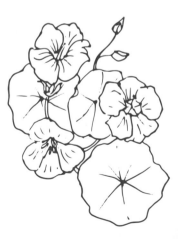

Sea vegetables, weeds, kelp
Stinging Nettle (see p. 160)
Watercress

SOUR

Pucker up! Sour-tasting remedies have an important role in the herbal world too. Much like bitterness, sour function helps us detect acids from rotting foods that could harm us. It can also be a great indicator of important nutrients – namely vitamin C and other antioxidants. The way our bodies react physiologically to sour herbs can have even more perks, such as preventing infection or pathogens, tightening tissues, and drying up excess fluids in the body. Like the salty taste function, sour helps hydrate and balance electrolytes. It boosts saliva flow for enhancing digestion while also promoting sweating.

Topically, sour can have astringent effects that are fantastic for skin, and this astringency can also help enhance anti-microbial or antiseptic effects, making them excellent herbs for topical wound care or oral care. Across the board, herbalists agree that the sour flavour is drying and cooling. Overall, sour herbs may have the most utilitarian healing functions of all: protecting against infection, fighting pathogens, promoting fever, cooling the body, and nourishing and tonifying the digestive system, tissues and skin.

Agrimony (see p. 99)
Blackberry
Citrus (juice)
Crampbark
Cranberry
Elderberry
Hibiscus
Nopal cactus
Peach
Raspberry
Rhubarb
Rosehips
Sumac (see p. 166)
Usnea

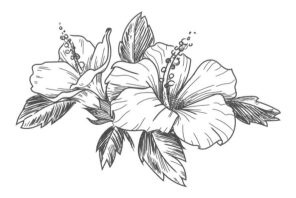

SPICY / PUNGENT

While not an official 'taste' per se, spicy and pungent herbs are a force to be reckoned with. They have one strong affinity over all: and that is with the heart, blood and entire cardiovascular system. Undeniably warming, spicy or pungent herbs (sometimes called 'acrid' herbs) can be either damp or dry in nature but lean on the drier side of things. Their greatest ability is to bring blood flow to the skin and stimulate it throughout the body, enhancing what is called 'vasodilation'. These effects can have benefits to the respiratory system and help open up airways to ease breathing during coughs, colds, flus and other upper respiratory issues. They're also known to give a substantial immune boost to the body.

Garlic (see p. 123)
Ginger
Horseradish
Hot peppers (cayenne, habanero, etc.)
Leek
Mustard (seed and spicy greens)
Onion
Shallot

AROMATIC

Also not an official flavour profile, aromatics are nevertheless important taste sensations – and fragrances – for healing. All the most popular selections for essential oils are aromatic herbs. You can identify them by their distinct flavours and aromas, hence their name. They can either be cooling or warming, but are almost always drying.

These herbs' powerful imprints on the senses (often making them a favourite for culinary arts or aromatherapy) are thanks to compounds called 'volatile oils'. A common hallmark of volatile oils is strong anti-microbial action, meaning the herb helps kill bacteria, fungi, and even viruses. It may also have some other specialized action: vasodilation, sedative action, anti-spasmodic (soothing cramps and muscle contractions), immune-boosting, and more.

Bee Balm (Monarda, Wild Bergamot)
Catnip
Cedar
Cinnamon
Kava Kava
Lavender
Lemon balm (see p. 133)
Lemon verbena
Mint

Oregano
Parsley
Pine (see p. 152)
Rosemary
Sage
Thyme

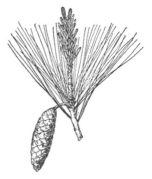

SAVOURY / UMAMI

Salty herbs are mineral rich, while sour could mean a treasure trove of hidden antioxidants and vitamins. Savoury, or 'umami' remedies – which don't tend to be classic herbs – are high in healthy fats, oils, proteins or other natural compounds that are fantastic targets for the brain and nervous system; lion's mane, shiitake and other medicinal gourmet mushrooms are the stars of the show here. Savoury remedies are generally inflammation-fighting, immune-boosting and nourishing as well as being nerve tonics or 'nootropic' (mushrooms specifically). They are also cooling and moistening, as a rule.

Nuts (especially avocado, walnut, chestnut etc.)
Lion's mane (see p. 139)
Maitake
Puffball mushroom
Shiitake

INDEX

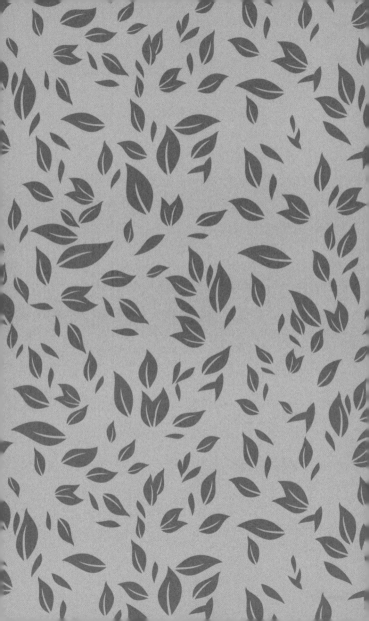